Chris Carmichael's
Fitness Cookbook

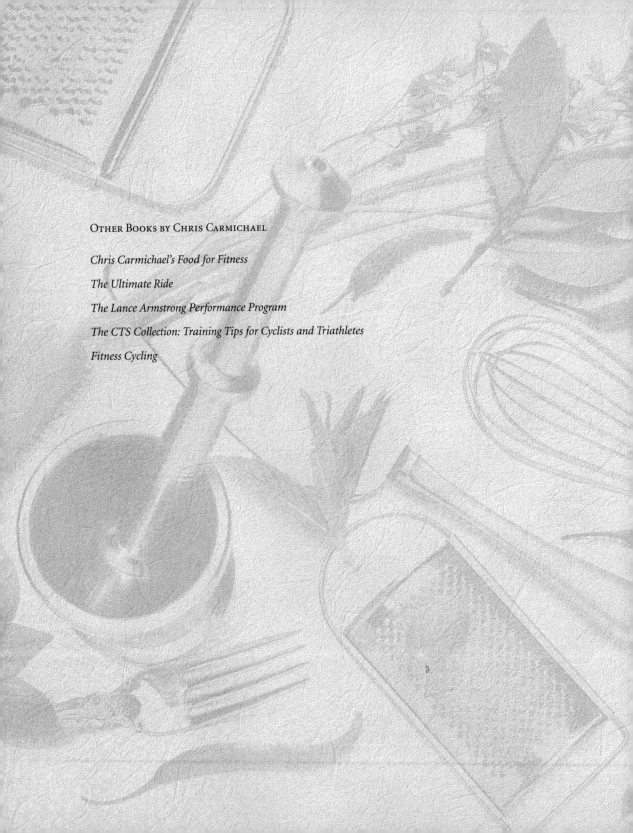

OTHER BOOKS BY CHRIS CARMICHAEL

Chris Carmichael's Food for Fitness

The Ultimate Ride

The Lance Armstrong Performance Program

The CTS Collection: Training Tips for Cyclists and Triathletes

Fitness Cycling

Chris Carmichael's

Fitness Cookbook

Delicious Recipes
for Increased Fitness,
Enhanced Health,
and Weight Loss

CHRIS CARMICHAEL
with JIM RUTBERG

Recipes by MARK TARBELL

G. P. PUTNAM'S SONS

NEW YORK

G. P. PUTNAM'S SONS
Publishers Since 1838

Published by the Penguin Group
Penguin Group (USA) Inc., 375 Hudson Street, New York, New York 10014, USA ·
Penguin Group (Canada), 90 Eglinton Avenue East, Suite 700, Toronto, Ontario M4P 2Y3, Canada
(a division of Pearson Penguin Canada Inc.) · Penguin Books Ltd, 80 Strand, London WC2R 0RL,
England · Penguin Ireland, 25 St Stephen's Green, Dublin 2, Ireland (a division of
Penguin Books Ltd) · Penguin Group (Australia), 250 Camberwell Road, Camberwell, Victoria 3124,
Australia (a division of Pearson Australia Group Pty Ltd) · Penguin Books India Pvt Ltd,
11 Community Centre, Panchsheel Park, New Delhi–110 017, India · Penguin Group (NZ),
Cnr Airborne and Rosedale Roads, Albany, Auckland 1310, New Zealand (a division of Pearson
New Zealand Ltd) · Penguin Books (South Africa) (Pty) Ltd, 24 Sturdee Avenue, Rosebank,
Johannesburg 2196, South Africa

Penguin Books Ltd, Registered Offices:
80 Strand, London WC2R 0RL, England

An application to register this book for cataloging has been submitted to the Library of Congress.

ISBN 0-399-15292-X

Printed in the United States of America
10 9 8 7 6 5 4 3 2 1

This book is printed on acid-free paper. ∞

BOOK DESIGN BY TANYA MAIBORODA

The information in this book is meant to supplement, not replace, proper nutrition and athletic training. The authors and publisher advise readers to take full responsibility for their safety and know their limits. Before practicing the methods and/or skills described in this book, be sure that your equipment is well maintained, and do not take risks beyond your level of experience, aptitude, training, and comfort.

The Periods, Carrier Method, and Carmichael Nutrition Program identified within this book are copyrighted works of CTS, Inc. No reproduction of this material is permitted without the express written permission of Carmichael Training Systems, Inc. Contact CTS at www.trainright.com.

The recipes contained in this book are to be followed exactly as written. The publisher is not responsible for your specific health or allergy needs that may require medical supervision. The publisher is not responsible for any adverse reactions to the recipes contained in this book.

While the authors have made every effort to provide accurate telephone numbers and Internet addresses at the time of publication, neither the publisher nor the authors assume any responsibility for errors, or for changes that occur after publication. Further, the publisher does not have any control over and does not assume any responsibility for author or third-party websites or their content.

Dedicated to parents whose healthy lifestyles provide our children
with positive examples of good nutrition, exercise, and balance

ACKNOWLEDGMENTS

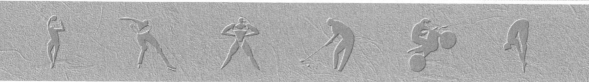

CHRIS CARMICHAEL

Putting this book together was a lot of fun, so much more so because of the skilled and supportive team I had the pleasure of working with. It has been great to collaborate with a world-class chef like Mark Tarbell. The recipes he and his team prepared for this book are exquisite, yet simple enough to be prepared by anyone, in any kitchen. Of course, I'd like to thank Sheryl Crow for making the introduction. My thanks also go to the photographers, John Rae and Paul Markow, for producing the photos. Closer to home, I'd like to thank all the people who helped bring this idea to fruition. Thank you to Jim Rutberg and Kathy Zawadzki for their ongoing contributions to my nutrition and wellness projects, and to Rhonda Mayo for her creativity in developing graphics for this book. My thanks also go to Lance Armstrong; we've come a long way together. My gratitude and love go to—more than anyone—my family, to Paige, Anna, and Connor.

MARK TARBELL

I'd like to thank Rick Purcell for introducing me to Sheryl Crow, then to Chris Carmichael years later. Thank you to Anne Ballman for all the testing and editing, and for keeping the recipes organized and on track. I couldn't have done this without you. Thank you to Jim Gallen for running Tarbell's and The Oven while I holed up and wrote. Thank you to Chef Paul Steele and Chef Josh Drage for sourcing ingredients, to Paul's wife, Kara, for testing recipes, and to Jody Knight for talking me into going to Aspen and for opening your home to me. Finally, thank you to Koschka for years of support, to my bike for keeping me sane, and most of all to Mom, Dad, Sis, Bro, and Red for the good stuff.

JIM RUTBERG

My thanks go to Chris Carmichael for his constant support and leadership, and to Mark Tarbell and his team for providing excellent recipes and photos. I'd also like to thank Kate Gracheck, Kathy Zawadzki, and Ashley Kipp for their help generating the nutrition information for the recipes. Above all, my greatest thanks go to my wife, Leslie. Thank you for your support during the long days and late nights that always accompany big projects.

CONTENTS

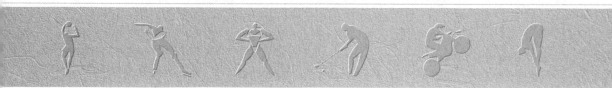

INTRODUCTION

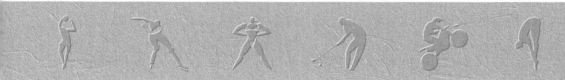

FOLLOWING THE RELEASE OF MY PREVIOUS BOOK, *FOOD FOR FITNESS,* I DID what naturally comes after the release of a new book: I went on tour. Obviously, the point of a book tour is to meet readers, sign autographs, and hopefully sell more books, but I've also found that book tours provide a great opportunity to listen to what the public wants most. People were receptive to the idea of matching their nutrition program with their exercise level, to letting their active lifestyle be the driving force behind the nutrients they chose to provide their bodies. They appreciated someone speaking directly to their segment of the population, rather than having to extrapolate the possible ways the newest fad diet and weight-loss program could be manipulated to meet their needs. Yet, in the midst of talking to people who enjoyed the book, and some who didn't, I realized I needed to take some of the ideas in *Food for Fitness* a step further.

Food for Fitness examined the reasons some foods provide better fuel than others, and why that is important for maintaining a healthy and active lifestyle. There were extensive lists of foods that were high-quality sources of energy, vitamins, minerals, and antioxidants.

We introduced the Carmichael Nutrition Program, applying to nutrition the concept of periodization in order to segment the year into four distinct periods, each with its own unique combinations of carbohydrate, protein, and fat recommendations. To take the information one step further, and to answer a recurring question from readers, I identified key foods that should be included in your nutrition program during each one of the periods.

Of course, the next step was to find a way to get this information out to the reading public; I again reflected on the interactions I've had with readers to guide my decisions. Many active people told me the recipes in *Food for Fitness* had breathed new life into their dull routines that had previously consisted of the same five meals, and they asked when they could expect to see more recipes. As sometimes happens, if you're fortunate, the ideas for a new project, and the people who could best bring them to fruition, converged one night in Aspen, Colorado.

It was just weeks after the 2004 Tour de France and the release of *Food for Fitness*. After becoming the first man to win the Tour six times, Lance had been traveling all over the map for media appearances and we hadn't talked much in a few weeks. We are so involved with each other's lives during the months prior to and during the Tour de France that we need to take a break from each other after it's over.

When he called me on an August afternoon, my first thought was, "He's early." He normally doesn't want to talk about training or the plan for next year until sometime in October. He was relaxed and easier to talk to than he had been in months, but that's what tends to happen when the pressure of winning the Tour is lifted. He told me Sheryl Crow had an upcoming concert in Aspen, Colorado, that he was going as well, and that I should bring the family and join them.

It wasn't until then that I realized I hadn't taken a day off since I left Colorado Springs for France at the end of June. I quickly agreed to join Lance and Sheryl in Aspen, and my wife and I decided to use the concert as the first stop on a much-needed weeklong family vacation.

The concert was terrific, and I was very happy to be there with my immediate family and several members of my extended family of Carmichael Training Systems coaches and staff who also made the trip. Lance and Sheryl had provided backstage passes, and I found it interesting to see Sheryl in her element. In what appeared to me to be a chaotic environment, she was comfortable and welcoming.

While Sheryl and her band were finishing up their last set, and a few encores, my business partner and friend Michael Goldberg, Lance, and I talked about the various dinner choices available in Aspen, even though Lance and I already had our hearts set on Michael's sushi restaurant, Matsuhisa.

Always a generous man, Michael's invitations to this impromptu post-concert dinner quickly multiplied, and by the time we all arrived at the restaurant, the party occupied several tables. Sometime during dinner, Sheryl introduced me to Mark Tarbell, a world-renowned chef and owner of Tarbell's in Phoenix. Sheryl raved about his skill in the kitchen, and quickly pointed out he also had a passion for cycling and mountain biking.

As Mark and I talked, the conversation quickly moved to food, particularly the close relationship between eating and performance. Mark had read *Food for Fitness* and was already incorporating the book's concepts into recipes served in his restaurant. I mentioned some of the ideas I'd been having about a follow-up book to *Food for Fitness,* and he expressed a keen interest in contributing his expertise to the project.

I wish I could say I put the project on the back burner for the next week while on vacation with my family, but that's not the way I work when I'm excited about a new project. By the time we arrived back in Colorado Springs, I'd already developed most of the plan for this book, including background information on Mark. Though I was immediately confident in Mark's ability, Sheryl confirmed he was a good guy who was reliable, a stickler for health and nutrition, and always exceeded expectations.

Through the following months, as the recipes started pouring in, I was constantly impressed with the creative and thorough approach Mark brought to the project. There often seems to be a trade-off between health and taste in recipes; the healthier you make a recipe, the more bland and boring it tends to become. As Mark proved with the recipes in this book, you don't have to sacrifice taste to eat for health and performance.

Little does Mark know, this is just the beginning. The active community is hungry for information and has a deep appreciation for good food and performance nutrition. I don't exactly know what the next project will entail—maybe a new line of fresh foods or a chain of restaurants for active people—but I look forward to a long and fruitful collaboration with Mark Tarbell, his expert team of chefs, and the wonderful staff of coaches and nutritionists at Carmichael Training Systems.

ACTIVE EATING FOR ACTIVE LIVING

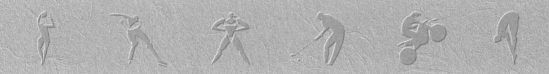

THERE HAS ALWAYS BEEN A STRONG CONNECTION BETWEEN FOOD AND EX-ercise, but much of it has been haphazard, anecdotal, and sometimes ridiculous. Centuries ago, some believed the key to being powerful was to eat the meat of a powerful animal, such as a bull. If you wanted to be fast, eat the meat of a fast animal, like a horse. More recently, there was a time when people believed athletes needed to eat eggs raw in order to get the full quality of their protein. As with all myths, there are kernels of truth in each of these ideas, but the relationships are wrong. Eating a bull won't make you powerful, nor will eating a horse make you fast, but consuming some high-quality cuts of red meat can help an athlete become both stronger and faster because of the protein and other beneficial nutrients the meat brings with it. More recently, we've realized that careful vegetarian athletes can obtain the same beneficial nutrients without including the red meat at all. With the knowledge we have gained about the relationships between specific nutrients and their influences on performance, recovery, health, and longevity, we can now more accurately recommend a wider variety of foods that meet the true and changing nutritional needs of active adults.

Many coaches, trainers, dietitians, and nutritionists have applied the newest information in sports nutrition to the manufacture of supplements or engineered foods, but too few have focused on the positive impact real food can have on active people. During my time as an athlete and coach over the past thirty years, I've seen, tried, and researched thousands of supplements. Some of them work, many of them don't, but the biggest lesson I learned is that the foods that make up a person's meals and snacks have a greater impact on their health and performance than any supplement on the market.

What's more, real food has added, albeit ambiguous, advantages over supplements. Meals play an important role in our lives. They are the times when families and friends gather to share stories, experiences, and the news of the day. Relationships are built and sustained across tables laden with good food and conversation, and that's a component that no supplement can reproduce.

Of course, the impact foods have on health and performance can be positive or negative, making your decisions around foods critical to your well-being. As an active person, the effect food has on your athletic performance is an additional and important consideration. Foods that supply nutrients that meet the demands of your lifestyle help you feel energetic, powerful, and healthy, while other foods leave you feeling empty, dull, and unsatisfied. The big question is, with all the options available, how do we choose the foods that will enhance our lives?

The answer is not as complicated as it may seem, but it does require paying some attention to the principles of nutrition and exercise. This means taking the time to examine the energy demands you're placing on your body, and then planning your nutrition program to address those demands. While this process is exhaustively covered in *Food for Fitness*, it warrants a brief overview here as well.

Eating for Your Active Lifestyle

In the context of an active, athletic lifestyle, food has to be thought of in a new way. We have to move beyond thinking about food as the primary determinant of body weight and see it as the fuel that enables us to achieve our goals. I can't stand the old adage that you are what you eat. You're *not* what you eat, you're a combination of the things you eat, do, think, believe, and feel. When I'm working with Lance Armstrong to prepare him for the Tour de France, I am involved in every aspect of his life, from his training to his nutrition, his goals to his personal life. Achieving your goals and living a successful, enjoyable life is a matter of maximizing your potential in *every* aspect of what you do. A great training program integrated into a misguided life won't work, but when everything works together, you can achieve any goal you set for yourself.

Straight Talk About Calories

Nutrition and activity levels are inexorably linked, whether you're talking about performance or weight loss. It's misleading to promote the idea that what you eat doesn't matter as long as you only consume as many calories as you burn. The truth is, some foods provide better fuel than others, meaning they allow you to use more of their calories for clean-burning energy. Carbohydrates can burn hot and fast; foods readily broken down to ready-to-use carbohydrate (glucose) can efficiently provide clean-burning fuel. In contrast, burning lactose, a carbohydrate found in dairy products, is like trying to burn damp logs. It'll burn if the flame is hot enough, but it's troublesome and not your best first choice. The key foods identified in this book have been chosen because they are optimal sources of energy, and because they carry other beneficial nutrients with them.

Not All Calories Are Created Equal

It's also misleading to say that a calorie is a calorie, regardless of where it comes from. It's only after food is broken down to its simplest units, at the moment it is ready to be thrown into the metabolic fire—*then* a calorie is a calorie. In the process of getting from the grocery store to your cells, however, not all calories are equal. Some foods bring additional positive benefits along with their calories, while others bring either nothing or else ingredients that pollute your body and contribute to the onset of disease. Wholesome, unprocessed, or minimally processed foods bring vitamins, phytochemicals, minerals, and trace elements into your diet—nutrients you need and benefit from, but would miss out on by eating only bleached white rice, refined sugar, and imitation cheese spread (also available in an aerosol can). In developing the recipes for this book, I asked Mark Tarbell to meet two challenges: create recipes that utilize primarily whole foods, and keep the recipes simple and convenient to prepare. My staff and I have made every recipe in this book, and I am pleased to tell you he exceeded my expectations with every one.

The Concept of Periodization

Whether you're on a structured training program or just lead an active lifestyle, your activity levels change during the year. In its simplest form, periodization is just a term we use to categorize these distinct segments of the year. In its more structured form, periodization makes training goals less intimidating by breaking them into smaller, more readily achievable pieces. In this manner, we break the year into segments so your training and fitness progress through a planned series of steps.

I've been using periodization with Lance Armstrong and all of my athletes for years. One of the reasons my coaching methods have been more successful than other periodized programs is that I extend the concept into the athletes' nutrition programs. Different training periods require different fuel mixtures, and when the fuel matches your demands, you reap huge rewards. Think of it in terms of a race car: when I was coaching IndyCar driver Eliseo Salazar, he came to drive a race at the Pikes Peak International Raceway. We sat down to talk about his training and nutrition program and he said, "You know, it's like in the car. When we come here, to high altitude, we have to run a different fuel because the air is so thin. The car won't run fast here with the fuel from sea level." Likewise, the food you eat to power your aerobic workouts in the winter isn't the right fuel mixture to achieve the speed and power you want in the summer.

How Periodization Works

The primary role of periodization is to arrange workouts and nutrition so that you reach your goals. Though there are many philosophies of periodization, I break the year into four primary segments, known as the Foundation, Preparation, Specialization, and Transition periods. Each period has a broad training goal, and each month within the period is focused on training that contributes to achieving it. The benefit of periodization is that by training the components of fitness individually, you can make greater gains in each component, and subsequently, make huge gains in overall performance.

What Does Periodization Have to Do with Nutrition?

Since your activity level changes as you move from one period to the next, the amount of energy you burn changes as well. If you're eating the same basic number of calories all year, there is most likely a portion of the year when you are eating more food than you need. Likewise, there's almost certainly a portion of the year when your training burns more calories and demands more nutrients than you're consuming. As a result, the relationship between activity level and energy intake typically looks like the one shown in Figure 1.

People who consume a low-calorie, low-fat diet all year out of fear of gaining any weight tend to eat as if they are in the Transition Period or Foundation Period all year. During the most active portion of the year, however, their caloric intake is far too low to meet their energy demands. At the other end of the spectrum sits the athlete who eats like the Specialization Period lasts all year. He has no trouble meeting his energy demands during the most intense portion of his season, but he quickly gains weight through the Transition Period and spends most of the Foundation and Preparation periods struggling to lose it again.

By patterning your nutrition program to match your training, you eliminate periods of the year where your caloric intake and energy expenditure are vastly mismatched. Not only does this ensure you have energy when you need it, it also allows you to achieve and maintain a healthy and optimal weight during each period of the year, without having to deprive yourself of food or force yourself to exercise longer just to burn off excess weight. As your training addresses different goals in different months of the year, you need to make sure

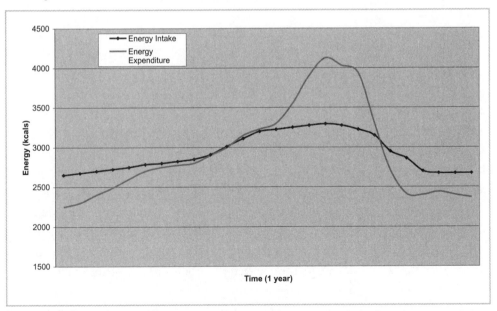

FIGURE 1: *Mismatched nutrition program. When the energy intake line is higher than the energy output line, you gain weight. When the energy output line is higher, you lose weight.*

you're eating the right amount, of the right kinds of foods, to support your workouts. Figure 2 shows the relationship between caloric expenditure and caloric intake when you apply periodization to your nutrition program.

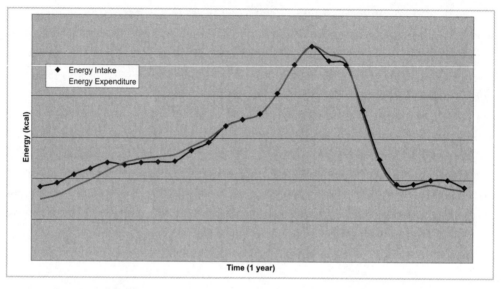

FIGURE 2: *Periodized nutrition program. Energy intake and expenditure track together across the year, eliminating periods of excessive weight gain or loss.*

Understanding What You're Burning and When You're Burning It

Matching calories consumed and calories burned is relatively easy, but in order to fuel a body optimally, you have to know what nutrients it's using for fuel, how much it's burning, and how quickly. It's important to realize that you burn carbohydrate, protein, and fat simultaneously whenever you exercise, regardless of the intensity of the workout. There is no such thing as an exercise that only burns fat, and there is never a condition where you can exercise effectively when you are totally depleted of carbohydrate, protein, or fat. Burning any one of these nutrients for energy requires the presence of the others.

Likewise, every time you exercise, you utilize all three of your primary energy systems: the immediate energy system, the anaerobic energy system, and the aerobic system. As the intensity of your workout changes, the percentage of your energy being delivered from each of these systems shifts; and with those shifts, there are changes in the amount of carbohydrate, protein, and fat being broken down for energy.

Several factors determine how cleanly your body operates. The foods you eat influence the availability of clean-burning fuels, and your fitness level influences the choices your body makes regarding which fuel to burn at what time. The cleanest way to burn fuel is with oxygen, using the aerobic system. The immediate energy system is pretty clean too, but it's not a major energy supplier. In fact, it can only supply energy for about 8–15 seconds of work. The anaerobic system is the real troublemaker, though. It's absolutely necessary, and the energy it supplies gives you the power to accelerate, sprint, and lift weights; but it's also a dirty, inefficient, smoke-belching, self-limiting system. That's why your training and nutritional choices should favor the development and use of your aerobic system: the clean, efficient, high-energy, unlimited energy system.

At low-intensity levels (20–35 percent of maximal effort), most of your energy is de-

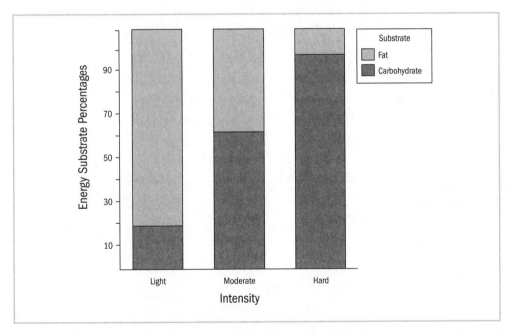

FIGURE 3: *The balance of fuel burned shifts to carbohydrate as exercise intensity increases. Adapted from* Energy Yielding Macronutrients and Energy Metabolism in Sports Nutrition, *edited by Judy A. Driskell and Ira Wolinsky (Boca Raton, FL: CRC Press, 2000), p. 22.*

rived from fat. In conditions where your body is depleted of carbohydrate, the rate at which you burn fat decreases, and your capacity for high-intensity exercise disappears. As the intensity of exercise increases to 35–50 percent of maximal effort, you're burning about a 50/50 mixture of fat and carbohydrate, and almost all of that fuel is being burned by the aerobic system. The percentage of energy derived from carbohydrate increases as intensity increases because you need energy more quickly than it can be liberated from fat. Interestingly, if it were possible to only burn fat for energy, you would be limited to exercise under 60 percent of your maximum effort.

The relative contribution of fat to energy production steadily decreases as exercise intensity moves from about 50 percent to 85 percent of maximal effort. This shift from deriving energy from a balanced mixture of fuels to burning much more carbohydrate occurs as you increase the amount of energy coming from the anaerobic system. Fat can only be burned through aerobic metabolism, but carbohydrate is burned aerobically *and* anaerobically, so the increased reliance on the anaerobic system to generate energy quickly leads to an increase in the total percentage of energy coming from carbohydrate, and a decrease in the percentage coming from fat. As your exercise intensity increases above 85 percent of maximum effort, the percentage of your energy coming from fat decreases even more, even though you're still burning some of the fat. It represents a lower percentage because you're burning so much more carbohydrate. The table below summarizes the relationship between intensity and fuel balance.

Approximate Percentage of Maximum Effort	Energy System(s) providing most of the energy	Approximate Balance of Fuel Use (Carbohydrate-Fat) (excludes small contribution from protein)
20–35	Aerobic	25–75
35–50	Aerobic	50–50
50–65	Mostly aerobic and little anaerobic	60–40
65–80	Aerobic and anaerobic	70–30
80–85	Mostly anaerobic and little aerobic	80–20
85–100	Anaerobic	>90–<10

As exercise intensity increases, the amount of energy coming from the anaerobic energy system rises, which in turn drives the shift to a greater reliance on carbohydrate fuel.

The Carmichael Nutrition Program

Nutrition and Training Across the Four Periods

Across all sports, I've seen the positive results athletes achieve when they pattern their nutrition program after their training. The concept is simple: when what you're burning for fuel and what you need for optimal performance change, you need to change your nutrition program accordingly. Over the years, I've found that applying the simple concept of periodizing nutrition provides my athletes with everything they need to train and compete at their best.

I focus on ensuring that an athlete gets enough carbohydrate and protein to meet his or her needs by relating the characteristics of the training period to the person's body weight. I end up with a prescription for a certain number of carbohydrate grams per pound of body weight along with a certain number of protein grams per pound of body weight. I then use these numbers, in relation to the four periods of the training year, to estimate their goal for total daily caloric intake. Fat ends up being the remainder of their calories after calculating carbohydrate and protein. I've made sure the amount of fat in this program, and in the recipes in this book, is relatively low, but not so low that people have to consciously spend time avoiding fat.

It is critical to remember, however, that the human body doesn't care about mathematics. Any number you calculate that is supposed to quantify what's happening inside your body or predict what it needs can only be regarded as an estimate. The numbers I calculate for my athletes, and the numbers you will undoubtedly calculate for yourself soon, are merely starting points. They may need to be adjusted up or down based on the details of your training program as well as your fitness and body weight goals. For many of the athletes I work with, especially the active fitness enthusiasts and amateur athletes, adjustments aren't necessary.

Determine Your Current Training Period

If you have not been training consistently and are just starting a training program, begin with the Foundation Period. Noncompetitive athletes, fitness enthusiasts, and active people sometimes have a little more trouble placing themselves in a training period. Historically, your training has remained the same all year, and most closely resembles Preparation Period Training. There is an aerobic component and an anaerobic component to your training, but neither receives enough attention to lead to significant progress. Essentially, you have a choice between placing yourself in the Foundation Period or the Preparation Period. If you're already in the most active portion of the year, you may want to place yourself in the Specialization Period for nutrition. Once your most active season is over, go straight into the Transition Period and progress from there. If you're uncertain, this is one of the times it is best to be conservative, which usually means starting with Preparation Period nutrition and adjusting as needed from there.

Carmichael Nutrition Program at a Glance

It is nearly impossible for anyone to doggedly adhere to fixed macronutrient intakes and percentages. It's not practical, or necessary, to weigh your food or preplan every meal so it has just the right amount of carbohydrate, protein, and fat. What's more, doing so would be to miss the bigger picture. There's nothing magical about eating 2.5 grams/pounds of carbohydrate or making protein 14 percent of your total calories. These things need to be viewed as details of a much more far-reaching concept.

Here are my nutritional guidelines:

Period	Carbohydrate		Protein		Fat	
	%	Grams/lb	%	Grams/lb	%	Grams/lb
Foundation	65	2.5–3.0	13	0.5–0.6	22	0.35–0.65
Preparation	65	3.0–3.5	13	0.6–0.7	22	0.55–0.65
Specialization	70	4.0–4.5	14	0.8–0.9	16	0.45–0.65
Transition	60	2.0–2.5	18	0.6–0.7	22	0.3–0.35

You can apply the numbers in the table above to yourself by multiplying the grams/pounds values by your body weight in pounds. I've provided two examples below:

For a 120-pound athlete:

Period	Total Calories	Carbohydrate		Protein		Fat	
		%	Grams	%	Grams	%	Grams
Foundation	1,800–2,200	65	300–360	13	60–75	22	45–55
Preparation	2,200–2,600	65	360–420	13	75–85	22	50–60
Specialization	2,700–3,100	70	480–540	14	95–110	16	50–55
Transition	1,600–2,000	60	240–300	18	75–85	22	40–50

For a 165-pound athlete:

Period	Total Calories	Carbohydrate		Protein		Fat	
		%	Grams	%	Grams	%	Grams
Foundation	2,500–3,000	65	410–500	13	80–100	22	60–75
Preparation	3,000–3,500	65	500–575	13	100–115	22	70–85
Specialization	3,700–4,200	70	660–740	14	130–150	16	65–75
Transition	2,200–2,700	60	330–410	18	100–115	22	55–70

Seeing the Bigger Picture

Look at the year as whole, starting with the Foundation Period, and you should see trends develop. For instance, your caloric intake follows the same trend as your training. Caloric intake increases as training volume and intensity increase during the Foundation, Preparation, and Specialization periods. It then falls during the Transition Period so you can restart the cycle. Following this general trend is more important than strictly increasing your carbohydrate intake from 2.5 to 3 grams/lb. Fat intake changes very similarly to the way total caloric intake changes. It is difficult to increase your caloric intake by eating more carbohydrate and protein but without eating any more fat. You can't be overly clinical when you think about nutrition, because that's not how you live your life. You eat full meals that contain a variety of foods, cooked in several ways. When you eat more food in order to get more carbohydrate and protein, your fat intake will naturally increase as well, and that's nothing to worry about or work to prevent.

Understanding the idea of periodization, the types of fuel you need to fuel your lifestyle, and the amount of food you should consume during each period is just part of the total equation. The critical step is to select foods that will enhance your active lifestyle. There are so many choices in supermarkets and restaurants that making good selections can seem daunting or overwhelming. Yet, if you ask some simple questions about the foods you're picking off the shelf or the menu, you can make the right choices every time.

The Carrier Method

I look at foods as vessels carrying supplies for the body. This is helpful because it illustrates that nutrients are not eaten in isolation. You may choose a food because you're after the carbohydrates it contains, but you're not just eating the carbohydrate portion. When you eat the entire food, you get everything else (the good and the bad) that it's carrying. When you look at foods in this light, it is relatively easy to group them into three categories: quality carriers, empty carriers, and pollutant carriers.

Quality carriers are the nutritional equivalent of the motor yacht: powerful, impressive, and stocked with amenities. Empty carriers are more like your standard rowboat: a no-frills, unrewarding, and inefficient way to get where you're going. Finally, the pollutant carrier is essentially a garbage barge: a vessel whose cargo does you more harm than good. The table below shows some examples of foods that fit into these three categories:

Carrier	Quality Carriers "Motor Yacht"	Empty Carriers "Rowboat"	Pollutant Carriers "Garbage Barge"
Additional cargo*	Vitamins, minerals, phytochemicals, antioxidants, fiber	Minimal amounts of beneficial nutrients beyond	High amounts of harmful pollutants, including saturated fat, trans fat, excessive sodium
Food examples	Spinach	Cola	Pork rinds
	Whole-grain cereal and bread	Low-fat candy (e.g., Pixie Sticks)	High-fat candy (e.g., Chunky Bar)
	Salmon	Kool-Aid	Doughnuts
	Sweet potatoes	Pretzels	Lard
	Kiwifruit	Low-fat cookies	French fries
	Chicken breasts	Iceberg lettuce	Fried chicken
	Brown rice	White rice	High-fat meats (pork ribs)
	Soy milk		

* Each individually listed food may not contain all of these additional nutrients.

The next big question, however, is: how do you tell what category your food choices fit into?

Nutrient Density

A nutrient-dense food supplies many beneficial components per calorie, allowing that food to have the greatest positive impact on your health and performance. Foods that are less nutrient dense aren't necessarily bad for you, but they're definitely less beneficial. A food's nutrient density can make the difference between its classification as a quality or empty carrier. Generally speaking, most fresh, natural foods are either quality carriers or empty carriers. This includes fresh fruits, vegetables, nuts, grains, and lean cuts of meat, chicken, and fish. Within these groups, however, some foods are more nutrient dense than others. The key foods that are highlighted in this book all fall into the nutrient-dense, quality carrier group.

Natural foods lose some of their quality and start heading toward the pollutant carrier category as they are processed into convenience-oriented, prepackaged foods. For instance, a fresh peach is a quality carrier because it supplies a lot of nutrients for the total calories it contains. In the process of being cooked, peeled, and canned in heavy, sweetened syrup it becomes an empty carrier food because the number of calories drastically increases and the nutrient concentration decreases, thereby reducing the food's ratio of nutrients to calories.

Many quality carriers are doomed to the pollutant carrier category by the ways they are cooked. A lean cut of red meat, like an eye of round steak, is a quality carrier because it is a great source of protein, zinc, and iron. Grilled, it remains a quality carrier, but breaded and fried on the way to making chicken-fried steak, it quickly becomes a pollutant carrier food. The same is true of chicken when it is served as fried chicken, and potatoes, onions, and other vegetables that are commonly deep-fried. The preparation methods used in the recipes you'll find in the following chapters have been carefully chosen to either reduce, or at least avoid adding, components that reduce the quality of the nutrients in the ingredients.

How to Use This Book

The remainder of this book has been divided into sections that focus on each of the four training periods of the year: the Foundation, Preparation, Specialization, and Transition periods. Within each section, the recipes feature one or more foods that are optimal sources of energy, vitamins, minerals, and antioxidants for the level of activity you are sustaining during that period of the year. That being said, variety is one of the most important components of a good nutrition program, and any of these recipes would be good options at any time of the year. Cold-water fish, such as salmon and tuna, are featured as key foods in the Foundation Period because they are great sources of complete protein and heart-healthy omega-3 fatty acids. The recipes in the Specialization Period tend to be higher in carbohydrate because of the increased intensity of exercise during this time of year, but the nutrients from salmon or other cold-water fish are still beneficial in the Specialization Period. By identifying a food as being key for one period of the year, I am not implying it is a poor choice during the other three periods. Rather, while all the foods identified in this book are great for your health and performance, some are best suited to meeting the energy and nutrient demands of a particular activity period.

Using Nutrition Icons

The recipes in this book have already been chosen for the positive impact their ingredients have on health and performance, so choosing the best among them is like choosing your favorite child. In order to help you choose the most appropriate recipe for your changing needs and desires, I devised a system of quick-reference icons you'll find on the top corner of recipe pages. I've found these icons to be useful because they provide context to detailed nutritional data and because a chart full of numbers doesn't give you the whole story.

Take, for instance, the fat content of a salmon recipe. Since salmon has no carbohydrate, all the calories come from protein and fat; and since it lives in cold water, salmon is regarded as a fatty fish. Listing the macronutrient composition of a salmon recipe might indicate that 40–50 percent of the calories come from fat, and I'd be hard-pressed to find a single athlete willing to eat anything that's 50 percent fat. What the numbers don't say, however, is that the fat in salmon is primarily unsaturated and rich in essential omega-3 and omega-6 fatty acids. The numbers don't tell you that populations that eat at least eight ounces of salmon or similar fish per week have lower incidence of heart disease and stroke. What's more, the absolute amount of fat in the recipe is not high, but it represents a high percentage of calories based on the absence of carbohydrate.

All the recipes in the following chapters use quality-carrier ingredients to create nutrient-dense final products, so you can't really go wrong preparing any one of them. At the same time, each recipe has specific characteristics that led me to select it for inclusion in this book. I've used the icons to highlight these features so you can quickly find recipes that are high in carbohydrate or rich in antioxidants, best for postworkout recovery, or a combination of these characteristics.

Firestarter

In the hours prior to your workouts, you want to eat foods that are easily digested and provide ready-to-burn energy. Preworkout meals should leave you feeling satisfied, but they shouldn't be so heavy that you feel sluggish and bloated when you start training. Recipes that carry this icon are high in carbohydrate, including both simple and complex forms. They also contain some protein, fat, and fiber, but are not high in any one of them, in order to keep the recipes light and energizing.

 Rapid Replenisher

After your workouts, the foods you eat have to be satisfying, rich in carbohydrate to replenish depleted energy stores, and rich in protein to build and repair muscle and maintain the immune system. Your body is most efficient at moving carbohydrate and protein into muscle cells within the first hour after exercise, and these recipes provide the nutrients your body needs to recover from today's effort and prepare for tomorrow's. The meals that tend to include these recovery foods tend to sit somewhat heavily in the stomach, which makes them very satisfying, but can also make them less desirable as preworkout meals. Recipes that carry this icon are good to eat after your workouts because of the ways they enhance your recovery and replenish depleted energy stores.

 Primary Fuel

Quite simply, carbohydrate is the primary fuel for performance, and recipes with this icon supply a great deal of this clean-burning nutrient. Look for this icon when you want a recipe that will supply 30 or more grams of carbohydrate per serving.

 Building Block

Protein provides the building blocks for every tissue in the body, and it also plays a huge role in maintaining your immune system. Recipes with this icon not only contain a large amount of protein (15 or more grams per serving), but also the protein is of very high quality. In cases where the protein source is from animal products, dairy, and/or soybeans, it is complete protein that contains all the essential amino acids.

Heart-Healthy Fat

For a long time, fat has been the nutrient everyone loved to hate, but a closer look shows it to be a necessary component of a balanced and high-performance nutrition program. During aerobic exercise, up to half the energy you burn can come from fat, and even at high-intensity levels, you're still burning some fat for energy. Fat plays an important role in cell walls, immune function, and reproduction, so eliminating it from your diet is not wise.

The healthy way to go is to moderate your fat intake and focus on mono- and polyunsaturated fats while limiting your intake of saturated fat. Foods like nuts, avocados, olive oil, and fish contain mono- and polyunsaturated fats, which have been shown to reduce your risk of heart disease, especially when they displace saturated fat intake. Foods that are quality carriers for fat also bring vitamins, minerals, phytochemicals, and fiber with them.

While your body can make most of the fatty acids it needs, it cannot make either omega-3 or omega-6 fatty acids. Obtaining these essential unsaturated fatty acids from food is beneficial because they have been shown to reduce your risks of heart attack and stroke, partly because they act to slightly reduce clotting in blood. The primary sources of omega-3 and omega-6 fatty acids are cold-water fish, flaxseed, flaxseed oil, soybeans, and canola oil. Recipes that are rich in heart-healthy fats, and low in saturated fat, will carry this icon.

 Cleanup Crew

Free radicals are a fact of life, even more so for active people and those living with air pollution. These rogue molecules damage cells throughout the body, and have been implicated in many diseases associated with aging. Since the energy-production centers of your muscles, the mitochondria, are particularly vulnerable, free radicals have been suggested as one of the primary causes for the diminished ability to produce energy associated with aging.

Antioxidants are your natural defense because they neutralize free radicals, minimize the formation of new ones, and repair the damage they've already caused. These helpful vitamins and minerals may not improve your athletic performance today or tomorrow, but they may play a big role in your long-term health and vitality. Foods rich in antioxidants include those rich in beta-carotene and other carotenoids, vitamins A, C, and E, and the minerals zinc and selenium. Recipes carrying this icon contain significant amounts of vitamins with antioxidant properties.

Healthy Snack

Sometimes you just want a good, healthy, energizing snack when you get home, in between classes, or for the road. To make finding these snacks quicker and easier, we gave them an icon of their own. Replace your soda-and-a-candy-bar snack with one that delivers the energy you need and a whole lot of nutrients you really want.

 Fiber

Even though fiber is a major component of a wide variety of fruits and vegetables, most Americans fail to meet the National Cancer Institute's recommendation of consuming 25–30 grams of fiber every day. Meeting this requirement goes a long way toward protecting you from several types of cancer, promotes regularity, and makes meals and snacks more filling. By making foods more filling, fiber can play a significant role in controlling caloric intake during the Transition and Foundation periods.

Choosing Your Servings

The recipes in this book have been created to produce four servings, and we have included the nutritional information for the recipes based on a single serving size. Part of the reason we provided the nutritional information for each recipe is to give you the opportunity to fine-tune your portion sizes. There may be times, especially during periods of high-intensity or high-volume training, when you may want to, or need to, eat one and half servings of a recipe rather than one. Likewise, there may be portions of the year when you want to reduce the portion size because you're not as active. We provided the nutritional information so you can determine how these changes will affect your intake of carbohydrate, protein, and fat.

Although you can use the recipes in this book to create entire meals, it is most likely that you will be combining a recipe from this book with other components to make up a complete meal. As such, it's important to have an idea of appropriate portion sizes for athletes. Since many athletes eat one and a half times the calories per day as sedentary people, it makes sense that you're going to be putting larger portions onto your plate. However, this larger portion size is not a license to blindly heap food onto your plate. The following table provides some reference points to help athletes determine appropriate portion sizes:

Food	USDA Serving Size	Looks like . . .	Normal Athlete's Portion	Looks like . . .
Cooked oatmeal, rice, pasta	½ cup	Ice-cream scoop	1–1.5 cups	An adult man's fist
Dry cereal	1 cup	1 large handful	1–1.5 cups	2 medium handfuls
Breads	½ bagel 1 slice of bread ½ pita pocket	N/a	1 bagel 2 slices of bread 1 pita pocket	N/a
Beans and legumes (peas, lentils, black beans, pinto beans)	½ cup	Ice cream scoop, lightbulb	1–1.5 cups	An adult man's fist
Nuts	⅓ cup	One handful	⅔ cup	Two handfuls
Meats	3 ounces	Deck of cards, palm of your hand	4–8 ounces	Checkbook, palm plus half of fingers
Fruit	1 medium-sized fruit 1 cup cut-up fruit	One baseball, clenched fist	1 large fruit, 2 medium fruits 1 cup cut-up fruit	Hand clasped around baseball
Peanut butter and similar foods	2 tablespoons	One golf or Ping-Pong ball	2–3 tablespoons	One racquetball

Other visual cues for determining portion sizes include:

- One teaspoon is about the same size as the end of your thumb.
- There are 3 teaspoons in 1 tablespoon, or three thumb portions.
- One cup of lettuce is often about four large leaves.
- A 1-pint takeout Chinese food container holds 2 cups.
- A medium-sized baked potato is about the size of a computer mouse.
- One ounce of cheese is about the size of your entire thumb.
- A standard serving size for a pancake is about the size of a CD.

Notes from the Chef

As a world-class chef, Mark Tarbell has the skill and experience to prepare some of the most complex meals you can imagine. That same intimate knowledge of food and cooking has allowed him to create great-tasting and healthy recipes that are simple enough for anyone to prepare at home. To make sure, we gave the recipes in this book to people no one would ever mistake for chefs, and asked them to prepare the recipes with tools they had in their own kitchens. Everyone had great results, and based on information they provided, Mark prepared some notes to help you create wonderful meals for yourself and your family.

Certain preparation instructions remain the same from recipe to recipe. Unless otherwise indicated, you should use the following instructions throughout the cookbook.

Leeks

Usually, recipes call for the white part of the leek only. The recipes in this book use the green part as well, since the leaves are full of vitamins. Unfortunately, the leaves are also like a rolled newspaper and trap a lot of dirt and sand inside. To prepare leeks for cooking, remove and discard 1 inch of the green tops and ½ inch of the root end. Cut the remainder as specified in the recipe, then rinse very thoroughly in a colander and pat dry with paper towels before proceeding.

Carrots

Always peel carrots, then remove the tips and the roots before cutting in the style indicated in the recipe.

Onions

With both yellow and green onions, remove and discard the roots and tips. Peel yellow onions, then stand them on their root ends. Slice in half, and then slice each half into lengths or cubes, or dice, as the recipe specifies.

Green onions are sliced in "ringlets" unless otherwise instructed.

Recommended Equipment

To prepare many of the recipes in this book, I'd recommend having a food processor and a blender. Other equipment that will help you speed through the recipes includes:

- A large colander for rinsing greens (and leeks!)
- A salad spinner for drying greens

- A very large mixing bowl
- A medium-size strainer
- Several sets of measuring cups and spoons (or you'll be fine with one set, but you'll have to wash your equipment as you cook)
- A good chef's knife
- A pepper mill so you can use freshly ground pepper in the recipes
- A cheese grater
- A broiler-proof sauté pan (such as cast iron)
- An oven-proof skillet (such as cast iron)

Kitchen Basics

By keeping the following ingredients in your kitchen, you can reduce your grocery shopping to just picking up the fresh individual items needed for specific recipes. Whenever possible, use organic products—most grocery stores now stock them. When you purchase fresh produce and herbs, take a little time to look for organic ingredients grown by local farmers. The flavors are superior, organic farmers do not use herbicides and pesticides, and you'll be doing your community a service!

Oils/Vinegars/Sweeteners	Dairy	Seasonings	Miscellaneous
Canola oil	Unsalted butter	Chili powder	Chicken stock (Low salt, organic)
Olive oil	Nonfat sour cream	Ground cinnamon	Brown rice
Extra-virgin olive oil	Nonfat cottage cheese	Salt	Long-grain white rice
Red wine vinegar	Nonfat plain yogurt	Kosher salt	Low-sodium soy sauce
White wine vinegar	Fresh parmesan	Sea salt	Hot sauce
White vinegar		Ginger powder	Oat bran
Good balsamic vinegar		Cumin (seeds and ground)	Rolled oats
Brown sugar		Whole black peppercorns	Fruits/vegetables
Raw honey		Ground nutmeg	Yellow onions
Mesquite honey		Curry powder	Lemons
Molasses		Ground coriander	
Maple syrup		Cayenne pepper	

2

KEY FOODS AND RECIPES FOR THE FOUNDATION PERIOD

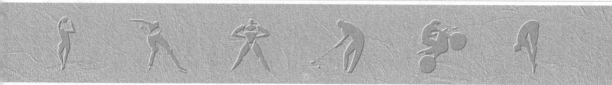

THE FOUNDATION PERIOD IS APTLY NAMED BECAUSE THE EXERCISE YOU perform during this time of the year lays the foundation upon which the rest of your training is built. The beginnings of a successful Specialization Period are established in the Foundation Period because this is the time when you focus almost entirely on your aerobic engine.

While we briefly reviewed the interaction between exercise intensity and the corresponding systems that provide energy for varying levels of activity, some people have the mistaken belief that the aerobic system shuts down once you start exercising at high intensity. People say they "go anaerobic," and believe it means they are getting all of their energy from the anaerobic system. The truth is, during high-intensity exercise, your aerobic system is working as hard as it possibly can, but since it can't meet your demands for energy quickly enough, the anaerobic system kicks in to fill the gap.

What does this mean for the Foundation Period, when most of your training is at relatively low-intensity levels? By building a stronger aerobic engine, you are effectively building a deeper and sturdier foundation. This allows your aerobic system to produce more of your energy at all intensity levels, including all-out efforts. You can think of the results in two ways. On one hand, more aerobic power means the anaerobic system kicks in later, and doesn't need to work as hard to supply the energy you demand at a given intensity. On the other hand, a stronger aerobic system allows the anaerobic system to kick in at a higher workload, which means its additional energy contribution allows you to go faster or perform at a higher level than you have before.

The training during the Foundation Period focuses on aerobic development and strength training. Improving the power and capacity of the aerobic engine requires workouts that overload the aerobic system for prolonged periods of time. This means doing endurance workouts that are longer and of moderate intensity. You might exercise at a level you can sustain for an hour or several hours with minimal interruptions. The key is to maximize the amount of energy you are deriving aerobically while minimizing the energy contribution from your anaerobic system.

The Foundation Period lasts about four months. For people living in the Northern Hemisphere and participating in primarily summer sports, this period usually occupies the late fall and winter months (November–February, give or take a month or two). For folks who want to be in the best shape for winter sports, the Foundation Period would occupy spring and early summer months (May–August, give or take a month or two).

Feeding the Foundation Period

From an energy standpoint, the Foundation Period is one of the less demanding portions of the year. The moderate intensity of your activities and workouts means the aerobic system can supply the vast majority of your energy. This is an important consideration for your nutrition program because it means you're burning a balanced mixture of carbohydrate, protein, and fat during exercise. It naturally follows that foods and meals you eat during this period should provide balanced amounts of these same nutrients.

Since the Foundation Period is not one of the most demanding portions of the year, it is often a time when active people consume many more calories than they need. As a result, people either tend to gain some weight during this period, or they have trouble losing weight they gained during the even less demanding Transition Period that immediately preceded it. It was for this reason that dietary fiber was one of my criteria for identifying key foods for the Foundation Period. Fiber is indigestible bulk found, in varying amounts, in fruits and vegetables. Because of its mass, fiber is filling, which means you can often keep caloric intake under control by increasing your consumption of high-fiber foods.

For people who are most active in the summer months, the Foundation Period usually falls within the coldest months of the year. This time of year is, coincidentally, the cold and flu season as well. Being active naturally strengthens the immune system, but the strain of exercise also places considerable stress on the immune system. It's not the exercise itself that makes a person more susceptible to infections, but the fact that exercise adds to the stresses your normal life already places on your immune system. If you're overworked, stressed at home, or staying up late studying, your training might add enough additional stress that it leaves you open to illnesses.

Fortunately, many whole foods contain compounds that reinforce your immune system, and incorporating these foods into your nutrition program may help you fight off colds, the flu, and more serious illnesses. Since the pathogens that cause these ailments are alive and well throughout the year, consuming foods that bolster your immune system are just as important for people who experience the Foundation Period during the spring and summer as well.

Key Foundation Period Foods

No single food has magical powers, so rather than provide three single key foods, I prefer to identify three groups of foods that should be incorporated into your Foundation Period nutrition program. In short, these are: bulbs, cold-water fish, and dried fruits.

Bulbs

While most people see images of tulips and amaryllis when they hear the word "bulbs," I'm not suggesting you eat flowering bulbs. Rather, I'm referring to vegetables like garlic, onions, leeks, and chives. While these ingredients are not going to be major sources of calories in your nutrition program, incorporating them into the meals you prepare may significantly impact your health and performance.

Organosulfides, the phytochemicals that give garlic, onions, leeks, and chives their characteristic (and pungent) odor, may play a role in preventing cardiovascular disease by lowering levels of LDL cholesterol (the bad kind) in blood. In truth, the studies conducted in this area don't conclusively support these claims, but evidence is still being collected and analyzed, and none of it shows these foods to increase your risk of developing cardiovascular disease.

Even though you might not consume pounds of onions or entire cloves of garlic, their addition to recipes brings vitamins A, C, and K without adding a lot of calories to the dish. Vitamins A and C have been shown to play a role in neutralizing and/or destroying free radicals within the body. Free radicals have been linked with oxidative stress, which may be a factor in aging and the typically detrimental effects aging has on athletic performance and health.

Relative to their caloric content, bulbs are also high in fiber. Again, you aren't going to obtain a huge proportion of your daily fiber intake from leeks or garlic, but considering that most Americans consume less fiber than they should every day, every little bit helps. Of the digestible portion of these ingredients, they are almost entirely carbohydrate and nearly devoid of fat.

Cold-Water Fish

Fish that live in cold water are fattier than tropical or temperate-water fish. While higher fat content is a bad sign in red meat, it makes cold-water fish a good choice because the fat is predominantly unsaturated and contains two heart-healthy essential fatty acids: omega-3 and omega-6. The cholesterol levels in fish are also lower than those in red meat and the dark meat portions of chicken and turkey. Populations that consume more of these fish have a lower incidence of cardiovascular disease, and in light of its effect on cardiovascular disease risks, the American Heart Association recommends eating at least eight ounces of cold-water fish per week.

Beyond the fact that fish like salmon, tuna, halibut, cod, and whitefish are good for your heart, they are also great sources of high-quality protein. Of the twenty amino acids that make up all the proteins in your body, eleven can be constructed inside your body. The remaining nine are referred to as "essential amino acids" because they have to be obtained from food. Fish is a source of "complete protein" because it supplies all twenty amino acids. The protein content of fish is roughly the same as that of red meat and poultry at 7 grams per ounce. A three- to four-ounce serving of fish is also rich in B vitamins, especially B_6 and B_{12}, thiamine, and niacin.

While fish supplies a host of beneficial nutrients, it does so without being excessively high in calories, making it a great addition to your Foundation Period nutrition program. Your muscles and immune system will benefit from the high-quality protein, your skin and cardiovascular system will welcome the omega-3 and omega-6 fatty acids, and your taste buds will enjoy some great meals.

One word of caution: although fish is a great source of protein and essential fatty acids, the FDA has issued guidelines for its consumption based on the presence of heavy metals, primarily mercury, in some species of fish. Women of childbearing age, and those who plan on becoming pregnant, should avoid four fish that contain especially high levels of mercury: shark, swordfish, king mackerel, and tilefish. In addition, tuna has been found to contain relatively high levels of mercury, and the FDA advises limiting your consumption of tuna, as well as other cooked fish, to 12 ounces or less per week. That's about 2½ cans of tuna, or 3–4 servings of fish.

Fish and Seafood (3-oz. serving, cooked unless noted, approx. 7 g protein/oz.)

Fish	Calories	Fat (g)	Saturated fat (g)	Monounsat. fat (g)	Polyunsat. fat (g)	Omega-3s (g)	Omega-6s (g)
Cod	90	0.7	0.1	0.1	0.2	0.14	0.03
Tuna	118	1.04	0.26	0.17	0.31	0.25	0.04
Halibut	119	2.5	0.35	0.82	0.8	0.47	0.18
Salmon	93	3.76	0.61	1.02	1.47	1.13	0.14
Tuna (raw)	122	4	1	1	1	0.195	0.031
Whitefish	146	6.38	0.99	2.18	2.34	1.57	0.54
Salmon (raw)	155	9	2	3	3	1.704	1.447

Frequently Dried Fruits

In light of the somewhat odd heading for this particular group of foods, it's probably best to get right to the items I'm referring to. The Foundation Period is a good time of year to include fruits like apricots, currants, dates, figs, raisins, and cranberries into your nutrition program. And while apricots, dates, figs, and cranberries are often eaten in their dried forms, they are good for you fresh, as well.

This group of fruits made the list of key foods for the Foundation Period because they are concentrated sources of carbohydrate energy. Handful for handful, they contain more energy than cookies, pretzels, or crackers. You'll find more energy in a handful of nuts, but a lot of the energy in nuts is coming from protein and unsaturated fat. In contrast, the energy from these fruits is almost entirely from carbohydrate. This is important because the Foundation Period represents an increase in activity level from the preceding Transition Period, but the increase in energy demand is not extraordinary. We're looking for ways to slightly increase your caloric intake, predominantly by increasing carbohydrate intake. Nuts and seeds, and the protein and fat they bring with them, play a more important role in the Preparation Period, where your total energy intake increases significantly.

In addition to carbohydrate energy, the fruits in this group are reasonably high in fiber, and deliver significant amounts of antioxidant vitamins and minerals. Figs, for instance, are high in beta-carotene, and currants deliver both vitamin C and the phytochemical lutein as part of their overall antioxidant contents. Lutein has shown promise in fighting free radical damage to tissues exposed to light, such as the skin and the eyes.

Oven-Roasted Garlic

SERVES 4
65 MINUTES

6 medium heads fresh garlic
2 tablespoons olive oil
1 teaspoon kosher salt

1 Preheat the oven to 350°F.

2 Cut the tops (opposite end of the roots) off the heads of garlic approximately one-quarter of the way down so that the garlic cloves are exposed. Discard the tops. Leave on the papery outside.

3 Place the garlic root-end down on a heavy baking sheet.

4 Sprinkle each head of garlic with the olive oil and salt.

5 Bake covered with foil for 35 minutes, then reduce heat to 300°F, remove the foil, and bake for 30 more minutes.

6 Remove from oven and set aside.

7 When still warm, squeeze out the garlic or scoop it out with a small spoon.

HINT: This can be spread on toast or crackers, stirred into a soup, added to warm pasta, or eaten on its own with a spoon. Store in refrigerator for up to 5 days in a closed plastic bag.

Nutrient	Calories (kcal)	Carbohydrates (g)	Protein (g)	Fat (g)
Single Serving	86	7	1	6

Leek and Rice Soup

  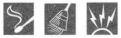

SERVES 4
1½ HOURS

6 stalks leeks, 1 inch of green tips and root ends removed,
    cut into ½-inch rounds.
1 quart plus 2 cups chicken broth
    (Vegan: Substitute vegetable broth.)
3 cups water
2 stalks celery, finely diced
1 medium carrot, cut into thin rounds
1 cup uncooked brown rice
Salt and pepper to taste
¼ cup Italian parsley
2 tablespoons extra-virgin olive oil
1 tablespoon fresh lime juice

1   Place all the ingredients except the parsley, olive oil, and lime juice in a 6-quart saucepan over high heat until boiling.

2   Reduce the heat to a simmer for 35 minutes.

3   Garnish with the parsley, olive oil, and lime juice and serve.

Nutrient	Calories (kcal)	Carbohydrates (g)	Protein (g)	Fat (g)
Single Serving	362	60	8	10

Chive Pesto on Whole-Wheat Toast Chips

SERVES 4
15 MINUTES

1 bunch fresh chives, root ends removed and discarded,
    cut into 1-inch pieces
1 teaspoon freshly squeezed lemon juice
3 tablespoons olive oil
1 tablespoon pine nuts
1 tablespoon grated Parmesan cheese
2 sprigs parsley, leaves only
Salt and pepper to taste
1 tablespoon water, in reserve to loosen the mixture
4 slices whole-wheat bread, cut into approximately 1-inch circles
    (Use a shot glass or some other small circular item;
    it should yield 16 circles.)

1   Place all the ingredients except the bread in a blender and purée until smooth, adding the 1 tablespoon of water if needed to make a thick creamy consistency; set aside.

2   Preheat the broiler on low setting, place the whole-wheat circles onto a small ungreased baking sheet, and toast until golden brown.

3   Top each toast circle with a small spoonful of the chive pesto.

4   Serve as an hors d'oeuvre.

Nutrient	Calories (kcal)	Carbohydrates (g)	Protein (g)	Fat (g)
Single Serving	154	12	4	10

Caramelized Onion Soup with Brown Rice

SERVES 4
45 MINUTES

1 tablespoon olive oil

1 large yellow or white onion, coarsely chopped

1 garlic clove, sliced into 5 pieces

1 tablespoon brown sugar

½ cup uncooked brown rice

1 tablespoon molasses

4 cups beef broth
  (Vegan: Substitute vegetable broth
  and add 1 tablespoon
  aged balsamic vinegar.)

2 cups water

1 tablespoon low-sodium soy sauce

½ cup red wine, port, or dry sherry; doesn't have to be fancy,
  just not "cooking" type wine

OPTIONAL GARNISH:

½ cup chopped fresh spinach or parsley

2 tablespoons currants

1 Place a 4-quart saucepan over medium heat.

2 When the pan is hot, add the olive oil and immediately add the onion. Stir until it begins to sizzle, then reduce heat to a slow sizzle, stirring often.

3 When the color of the onions begins to look a dark golden brown, add the garlic, molasses, rice, and brown sugar and cook for 2 minutes, stirring often.

4 | Add the remaining ingredients, turn heat up to high until it begins to boil, then turn down to a simmer.

5 | Adjust the heat to a high simmer and cook uncovered for 25 minutes, until the rice is puffed up and soft, stirring occasionally.

6 | Mix and stir in the optional garnish just before serving.

Nutrient	Calories (kcal)	Carbohydrates (g)	Protein (g)	Fat (g)
Single Serving	171	26	10	3

Warm Fig and Arugula Salad

SERVES 4
15 MINUTES

Good Basic Salad Dressing (page 65)

4 cups baby arugula (You can also use baby spinach, mizuna,
   or mustard greens—all these greens can be peppery.)

1 head butter lettuce, cleaned, dried, and torn into smaller pieces

8 fresh figs (substitute dried figs out of season),
   stems removed and discarded, cut in half

8 small shavings of Parmesan cheese,
   or 2 tablespoons grated Parmesan cheese

1 | Preheat the broiler on high setting.

2 | Stir all the dressing ingredients together in a small mixing bowl, and set aside.

3 | Place all the lettuce in a large mixing bowl.

4 | Place the fig halves on a small baking sheet and place under the broiler for 3–5 minutes, until warm and slightly browning, then turn off broiler.

5 | Mix the lettuce with enough of the reserved dressing to moisten the leaves.

6 | Arrange the lettuce on four salad plates with the warm figs and place the Parmesan shavings on top.

Nutrient*	Calories (kcal)	Carbohydrates (g)	Protein (g)	Fat (g)
Single Serving	105	21	3	1

*Good Basic Salad Dressing not included in these numbers.

Pan-Roasted Salmon with Caramelized Onion and Orange Sauce on Brown Rice

SERVES 4
1 HOUR

SALMON:

3 tablespoons olive oil

4 boneless, skinless salmon fillets (6 ounces each)

    (Vegan: Substitute four 4-ounce bricks fresh tofu,

    patted dry, seared in a hot nonstick pan with olive oil.

    Warm in a 400°F oven for 10 minutes before serving.)

1 tablespoon freshly squeezed lemon juice

½ teaspoon freshly ground black pepper

½ teaspoon salt

1   Preheat the oven to 400°F.

2   Warm a large sauté pan over medium-high heat.

3   Add the oil, wait 1 minute, then add the salmon or tofu.

4   Sear on one side for 5 minutes, then flip to other side for 1 minute.

5   Salmon: Roast in preheated oven for 10–20 minutes, until it begins to flake when pushed.

6   Tofu: Roast in preheated oven for 5–10 minutes, until warmed through.

7   Sprinkle with the lemon, salt, and pepper before serving.

CARAMELIZED ONION AND ORANGE SAUCE:

1 tablespoon olive oil

1 medium onion, sliced into thin strips

1 tablespoon brown sugar

1¼ cups freshly squeezed orange juice

¼ cup cranberry juice

1 tablespoon cold unsalted butter

1 | Place a 3-quart sauce pan over medium heat.

2 | Heat the oil for 1 minute, then add the onion and cook slowly for 10–15 minutes, stirring constantly until golden brown. Be careful not to burn.

3 | Add the brown sugar and stir for 2 minutes.

4 | Add the juices and simmer uncovered for about 15 minutes, until all but 4 table-spoons of the liquid is gone.

5 | Stir in the butter.

6 | Remove from heat and set aside to spoon over the top of the salmon.

HELPFUL HINT: If you don't have enough saucepans to do all this at once, make the onion mixture ahead of time and leave at room temperature up to 45 minutes. Place in the oven for 3 minutes at serving time.

BROWN RICE:

1 tablespoon canola oil

½ small onion, finely minced

1 cup uncooked brown rice

1½ cups water

Salt and pepper to taste

1 teaspoon freshly squeezed lemon juice

Zest of ½ lemon

1 | Place a 2-quart saucepan over medium-high heat.

2 | Add the canola oil.

3 | Add the minced onion and cook for 3 minutes, stirring constantly.

4 | Add the brown rice and cook, stirring, for 2 minutes.

5 | Add water.

6 Reduce to a simmer, cover, and cook for 15 minutes, until all the water is absorbed, stirring occasionally.

7 Remove from the heat, fluff up, and season with the salt, pepper, lemon juice, and zest to taste.

TO SERVE: Use the brown rice as a base. Place the salmon or tofu on top and spoon onion mixture over.

Nutrient	Calories (kcal)	Carbohydrates (g)	Protein (g)	Fat (g)
Single Serving	557	54	39	21

Roasted Halibut with Mediterranean Lentils and Olives

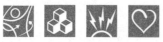

SERVES 4
2 HOURS

LENTILS:

1½ cups green lentils

3 cups cool water

½ large onion, cut into ½-inch pieces

5 garlic cloves, minced (3 for lentils, 2 for peppers)

3 sprigs fresh thyme

2 tablespoons olive oil (for tossing with the lentils after cooking)

8 green olives, pitted and cut into quarters

8 black olives, pitted and cut into quarters

Pepper and a little salt to taste (Note: The olives have salt.)

HALIBUT:

1 pound, 4 ounces halibut, skinned and cut into 4 equal portions
    (haddock or whitefish may be used instead)

1 tablespoon olive oil (for sprinkling on top)

Pepper and a little salt (on fish prior to searing)

1 teaspoon freshly squeezed lemon juice (for sprinkling on top)

1 sprig fresh thyme (to add aroma during cooking)

RED PEPPERS:

1 red bell pepper, cored, seeded, and cut lengthwise
    into ⅛-inch-thick strips

1 tablespoon olive oil

1 teaspoon freshly squeezed lemon juice

Pepper and a little salt to taste

1 | Place the green lentils in a medium mixing bowl, cover with warm water, and let stand for 30 minutes. This can be done in the morning before work. Then strain and rinse before beginning cooking.

2   Preheat the oven to 400°F for the halibut.

3   Place a 3- to 4-quart saucepan over medium heat. Add the lentils, onion, garlic, and thyme to the pan. Cook 30–40 minutes, until the lentils are slightly firm (not mushy and not grainy). Lentils should have a slight bite.

4   In a roasting pan, place the halibut, rubbed with olive oil, seasoned with salt and pepper (optional), and sprinkled with freshly squeezed lemon juice. Lay the thyme on the pan. Roast for 35–45 minutes. (If the halibut is 1 inch thick or less, cook for less time; if it is 1½ inches or more, cook for more time.) Remove from the oven and set aside.

5   Strain the lentils, remove the sprigs of thyme, place in a sauté pan over low heat, and toss with the 2 tablespoons of olive oil and the olives. Season with pepper and salt and set aside.

6   Place the bell pepper, 1 tablespoon olive oil, and lemon juice in a large sauté pan over medium heat. Cook for 30 minutes, stirring occasionally, and do not let it burn. Season to taste with the salt and pepper.

TO SERVE: Spoon the lentils in the center of the plate. Place the halibut on top of lentils. Cover top of fish with red peppers. Enjoy!

Nutrient	Calories (kcal)	Carbohydrates (g)	Protein (g)	Fat (g)
Single Serving	596	52	52	20

Oven-Seared Tuna with
Sweet Potato Mash and Chive Sauce

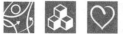

SERVES 4
1 HOUR

TUNA:

4 tuna steaks (6 ounces each)
   (Vegan: Substitute 4-ounce bricks of fresh tofu,
   patted dry, seared in a hot nonstick pan with olive oil.
   Warm in a 400°F oven for 10 minutes before serving.)
Salt and pepper
1 tablespoon olive oil, for sprinkling the top

1 Preheat the broiler on high setting.

2 Arrange the tuna steaks on a baking sheet.

3 Place under the broiler for 3 minutes.

4 Turn the steaks over and sprinkle with the salt, pepper, and olive oil.

5 Place back under the broiler for 5 minutes, or until cooked to the desired doneness.

NOTE: It's good to have a golden brown char to the top, and tuna is excellent when served reddish-pink in the middle. When well done it tends to be dry. Remove from broiler.

SWEET POTATO MASH (page 127)

This is also great over chicken or steak.

1 cup fresh spinach, leaves picked off and stems discarded.

2 ounces fresh tofu

3 tablespoons nonfat sour cream

    (Vegan: Add 2 ounces more fresh tofu.)

2 teaspoons freshly squeezed lemon juice

1 tablespoon olive oil

4 tablespoons grated Parmesan cheese

    (Vegan: Use soy provolone or Monterey Jack cheese, grated.)

1½ bunches fresh chives, cut into ½-inch pieces.

½ cup water

Salt and pepper to taste

1 Place the spinach, tofu, sour cream, lemon juice, olive oil, and Parmesan in a blender and purée until smooth.

2 Add the chives once the mixture is blended.

3 Add the water little by little and continue to blend until the sauce is pourable and smooth.

4 Season with the salt and pepper to taste.

TO SERVE: Arrange a pile of sweet potatoes on each plate. Place a tuna steak on top. Drizzle the sauce over the top.

Nutrient*	Calories (kcal)	Carbohydrates (g)	Protein (g)	Fat (g)
Single Serving	330	5	46	14

*Potato Mash is not included in these numbers.

Oven-Seared Tuna with Tomato Relish and Quinoa

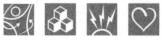

SERVES 4
40 MINUTES

TUNA:

4 tuna steaks
   (Vegan: substitute four 4-ounce bricks of fresh tofu,
   patted dry, seared in a hot nonstick pan with olive oil.
   Warm in a 400°F oven for 10 minutes before serving.)
1 tablespoon olive oil
Salt and pepper to taste

1 Preheat the broiler on high setting.

2 Arrange the tuna steaks on a baking sheet.

3 Place under the broiler for 3 minutes.

4 Turn the steaks over and sprinkle with the olive oil, salt, and pepper.

5 Place back under the broiler for 5 minutes, or until cooked to the desired doneness.

NOTE: It's good to have a golden brown char to the top, and tuna is excellent when served reddish-pink in the middle. When well done it tends to be dry.

TOMATO RELISH:

Also great for stirring into a warm pasta.

1 medium tomato, cored and cut into 4 pieces
6 large green olives, pitted
1 garlic clove, peeled and cut into 4 pieces
Leaves picked from 2 sprigs of fresh oregano, or 2 teaspoons dried oregano
3 tablespoons olive oil
1 teaspoon red wine vinegar
Salt and pepper to taste

1 Place all the ingredients in a food processor and process for 30 seconds, until the mixture is a rough-cut salsa.

QUINOA:

1 cup quinoa, rinsed in a strainer and dried

2 cups water

2 tablespoons olive oil

1 tablespoon freshly squeezed lemon juice

¼ cup currants

Salt and pepper to taste

1 Place the quinoa and water in a 2-quart saucepan over high heat.

2 Bring to a boil, then reduce to a medium simmer, cover, and cook for 12–15 minutes, until all the water is absorbed.

3 Remove from the heat, stir in the olive oil, lemon juice, currants, salt, and pepper, and fluff with a fork.

TO SERVE: Make a bed out of the quinoa, place tuna on top, and spoon tomato relish over.

Nutrient	Calories (kcal)	Carbohydrates (g)	Protein (g)	Fat (g)
Single Serving	595	33	46	31

Oven-Seared Cod and Caramelized Onions, Roasted Potatoes, and Crushed Parsley Sauce

SERVES 4
1 HOUR

COD:

4 codfish fillets (6 ounces each)

    (Vegan: Substitute four 4-ounce bricks fresh tofu,

    patted dry, seared in a hot nonstick pan with olive oil.

    Warm in a 400°F oven for 10 minutes before serving.)

3 tablespoons olive oil

Salt and pepper

1 Preheat the broiler on high setting and arrange the cod fillets on a baking sheet.

2 Place under the broiler for 4 minutes.

3 Turn the fillets over and sprinkle with the olive oil, salt, and pepper.

4 Place back under the broiler for 10 minutes, until the fillets just begin to flake when pressed with a fork.

NOTE: It's good to have a golden brown char to the top. It is important to cook cod through, as it will be more tender.

CARAMELIZED ONIONS (page 155)

ROASTED POTATOES:

These can be done a day in advance and reheated in a 400°F oven for 10 minutes.

3 medium russet potatoes, scrubbed,

    skins left on, and cut into 8 pieces

¼ cup olive oil

2 teaspoons salt

1 teaspoon pepper

1 | Preheat the oven to 450°F.

2 | Place the potatoes in a 3-quart saucepan with enough water to cover by 2 inches, and place over high heat.

3 | Boil until the potatoes are semisoft to the fork.

4 | Remove the pan from heat, and drain potatoes.

5 | Place the potatoes in a large mixing bowl and toss with the salt, pepper, and olive oil.

6 | Spread the potatoes on a baking sheet and bake for 15 minutes, or until golden brown.

CRUSHED PARSLEY SAUCE:

This is excellent with grilled pork, as well.

½ bunch parsley, finely chopped
1 garlic clove, finely minced
3 tablespoons olive oil
1 tablespoon freshly squeezed lemon juice
1 teaspoon chopped fresh thyme, or ¼ teaspoon dried thyme
Salt and pepper to taste

Place all the ingredients in a mixing bowl; stir and season, or place all the ingredients in a food processor and process into a rough chopped mixture.

TO SERVE: Make a base of the potatoes. Place the cod on top. Top with the caramelized onion. Drizzle with the parsley sauce.

Nutrient*	Calories (kcal)	Carbohydrates (g)	Protein (g)	Fat (g)
Single Serving	337	5	32	21

*Caramelized onions not included in these numbers.

Roasted Salmon with Spinach and Figs

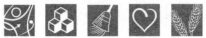

SERVES 4
25 MINUTES

4 boneless, skinless salmon fillets (6 ounces each)
    (Vegan: Substitute four 4-ounce bricks fresh tofu,
    patted dry, seared in a hot nonstick pan with olive oil.
    Warm in a 400°F oven for 10 minutes before serving.)
1 tablespoon olive oil
Salt and pepper to taste

1 | Preheat the oven 450°F.

2 | Arrange the salmon on a baking sheet.

3 | Sprinkle with the olive oil, salt, and pepper.

4 | Roast for 15 minutes.

5 | Turn the broiler on high setting.

6 | Place under the broiler for 4 minutes.

NOTE: It's good to have the salmon golden brown to the top. It is important to cook salmon through, as it will be more tender.

SPINACH AND FIGS:

3 tablespoons olive oil (substituting 1 stick unsalted butter will make it richer)
½ medium onion, peeled, trimmed, and cut into 10 even sections
1 pound fresh spinach, torn into smaller pieces (remove the large stems)
¾ cup dried figs, chopped into pieces
½ teaspoon ground nutmeg
Salt and pepper to taste

1 | Place a 4-quart saucepan over medium heat.

2 | When hot, add the olive oil or butter and the onion at the same time and stir constantly for 30 seconds.

3 | Turn heat down slightly, then cook for 2 minutes, stirring occasionally.

4 | Add the remaining ingredients and stir until spinach begins to soften.

5 | Remove from heat and season.

TO SERVE: Arrange plate with the spinach as base and salmon on top.

Nutrient	Calories (kcal)	Carbohydrates (g)	Protein (g)	Fat (g)	Total Dietary Fiber (g)
Single Serving	424	31	39	16	8

Penne Pasta Salad with Smoked Salmon, Spinach, and Basil

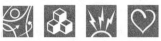

SERVES 4
30 MINUTES

10 ounces penne pasta

1 teaspoon salt

6 ounces smoked salmon, thinly sliced (see Note)

¾ cup fresh spinach, stemmed and torn into small pieces

¼ cup basil, stems picked off and leaves torn into medium-size pieces

2 tablespoons capers, drained

3 tablespoons olive oil

1 tablespoon and 1 teaspoon freshly squeezed lemon juice

Salt and pepper to taste

1 Place a 4-quart saucepan filled ⅔ with water and the 1 teaspoon salt over high heat.

2 Bring to a boil, then add the pasta.

3 Cook for 12 minutes, until the pasta has a little firmness but no raw flour taste. Test by removing one piece, set aside to cool, then taste.

4 Remove from the heat, drain, run cold water over the pasta to stop the cooking, and set aside to cool.

5 Place all the ingredients in a large mixing bowl, mix gently, and serve.

NOTE: Instead of smoked salmon, use 4 boneless, skinless salmon fillets (6 ounces each) and 1 tablespoon olive oil. Preheat the oven to 400°F. Place the salmon on a baking sheet rubbed with olive oil. Bake for 25–30 minutes.

Nutrient	Calories (kcal)	Carbohydrates (g)	Protein (g)	Fat (g)
Single Serving	360	44	19	12

Pan-Roasted Cod with Fork-Mashed Sweet Potatoes
and Green Olive, Lemon, and Chive Sauce

SERVES 4
40 MINUTES

COD:

4 skinless, boneless cod fillets (6 ounces each)

(Vegan: Substitute four 4-ounce bricks fresh tofu, patted dry,

seared in a hot nonstick pan with olive oil.

Warm in a 400°F oven for 10 minutes before serving.)

1   Preheat the oven to 400°F.

2   Place the cod fillets on a baking sheet.

3   Place in oven for 25–30 minutes, or until cooked to desired degree.

4   Place under the broiler on high setting for 3–5 minutes to sear the top.

FORK-MASHED SWEET POTATOES:

These can be served with almost anything.

2 small sweet potatoes, scrubbed and cut into 8 pieces

1 teaspoon salt

½ cup 1 percent milk

(Vegan: Substitute ½ cup plain soy milk.)

¼ stick unsalted butter

(Vegan: Omit butter.)

1 tablespoon olive oil

Salt and pepper to taste

1   Fill a 4-quart saucepan ⅔ with water and 1 teaspoon salt, set on high heat, and bring to a boil.

2   Add the sweet potatoes and cook for 15 minutes, until soft but not mushy.

3 | Remove from the heat, drain, and place back into the pot.

4 | Add the milk, butter, and olive oil and mash with a fork until well blended. (Depending on the size of the potatoes, you may need to add more milk.)

5 | Season to taste with salt and pepper.

TO SERVE: Place the mashed sweet potatoes on the plate first. Place the cod on top. Spoon the sauce all around.

COD ALONE:

Nutrient	Calories (kcal)	Carbohydrates (g)	Protein (g)	Fat (g)
Single Serving	274	5	32	14

MASHED SWEET POTATOES:

Nutrient	Calories (kcal)	Carbohydrates (g)	Protein (g)	Fat (g)
Single Serving	166	17	2	10

GREEN OLIVE, LEMON, AND CHIVE SAUCE:

Great when mixed in with fettuccine.

¾ cup green olives, pitted

1 bunch fresh chives, cut into 1-inch pieces

1 tablespoon parsley

2 tablespoons freshly squeezed lemon juice

1 teaspoon chopped fresh thyme, or ¼ teaspoon dried thyme

2 tablespoons olive oil

Salt and pepper (Note: Olives are salty, so little or no salt is needed.)

4 tablespoons water, set aside to create desired thickness of sauce

1 | Place all the ingredients except the water in a food processor and pulse until the mixture is in small pieces.

2 | Add the water to reach a spreadable consistency.

One-Pot Whitefish Chowder with Garlic and Potato

SERVES 6
1 HOUR, 10 MINUTES

½ bottle dry white wine, like Sauvignon Blanc

4 cups water

1 tablespoon freshly squeezed lemon juice

1½ tablespoons chopped fresh thyme, or 3 teaspoons dried thyme

1 medium leek, root end and 1 inch of green tips removed,
    outer layer discarded, sliced into 1-inch rounds

1 medium carrot, sliced into ¼-inch rounds

1 medium red or yellow bell pepper, cored, seeded, and cut into ¼-inch strips

1 large yellow onion, sliced lengthwise into 10 pieces

2 medium russet potatoes, scrubbed, skins left on, and cut into 8 pieces

10 ounces boneless, skinless whitefish or codfish, cut into 5 pieces

8 medium mussels or clams, cleaned and fresh

2 cups 1 percent milk

Salt and pepper to taste

1   Place all the ingredients except the fish, milk, salt, and pepper in a 5-quart saucepan over high heat.

2   When the liquid comes to a boil, turn down to a high simmer for 20 minutes.

3   Add the fish and milk, stir once, and bring back to a simmer for 5 minutes. Season to taste with the salt and pepper.

Nutrient	Calories (kcal)	Carbohydrates (g)	Protein (g)	Fat (g)
Single Serving	156	14	16	4

Atlantic Cod with Buttered Leeks and Brown Rice

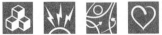

SERVES 4
35 MINUTES

COD:

4 medium leeks, root end and 1 inch of green tips removed,
    outer layer discarded, sliced into 1-inch rounds
1 stick unsalted butter
4 codfish fillets (6 ounces each)
    (Vegan: Substitute four 4-ounce bricks fresh tofu,
    patted dry, seared in a hot nonstick pan with olive oil.
    Warm in a 400°F oven for 10 minutes before serving.)
½ cup dry white wine, like Sauvignon Blanc (or substitute ½ cup water
    with 1 tablespoon freshly squeezed lemon juice added)
Salt and white pepper to taste

1 Place a wide 3-quart saucepan over medium heat, add the leeks and the butter, and stir until the butter has melted.

2 Place the cod fillets on top of the leeks. Add the wine and sprinkle a little salt and white pepper over the top. Cover with lid or foil, turn heat down to medium-low, and simmer for 17–20 minutes.

3 Uncover and let cook for another 3 minutes, until fish begins to flake when pressed with fingers.

RICE:

2 tablespoons unsalted butter
1 cup uncooked brown rice
1½ cups water
1 tablespoon low-sodium soy sauce
Salt and white pepper to taste

1   Place a 2-quart saucepan over medium-high heat. When hot, add the butter and the rice, and stir until the rice becomes a little translucent.

2   Add water and soy sauce, turn down to a simmer, cover, and simmer for 25 minutes, stirring occasionally.

3   When rice has no more liquid and tastes cooked, season it with salt and white pepper and fluff with a fork.

TO SERVE: Use rice as a bed, place the cod on top, and spoon the leeks over and around the cod.

Nutrient	Calories (kcal)	Carbohydrates (g)	Protein (g)	Fat (g)
Single Serving	516	49	35	20

Smoked Salmon and Chive Omelet

 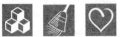

SERVES 2
15 MINUTES

2 tablespoons olive oil

2 large eggs and 4 large egg whites, beaten

3 tablespoons water

½ bunch fresh chives, cut into ¾-inch pieces

3 ounces smoked salmon

2 tablespoons nonfat sour cream mixed with 1½ teaspoons of water
to make the consistency easy to spoon over the finished omelet

Salt and pepper to taste

1 Place a medium-size sauté pan over high heat. When hot add the olive oil, then the eggs and half of the chopped chives.

2 Turn the heat down to medium-high and stir the eggs as if you're making scrambled eggs for 30 seconds to 1 minute.

3 Once 40 percent of the eggs are cooked, stop stirring.

4 Lay the smoked salmon on top and sprinkle the rest of the chives over the salmon.

5 Cover for 3–4 minutes on heat.

6 Remove the cover and place on a plate (omelet can be folded or left open-faced).

7 Stir water into sour cream and spoon over omelet.

8 Season to taste with salt and pepper.

Nutrient	Calories (kcal)	Carbohydrates (g)	Protein (g)	Fat (g)
Single Serving	266	11	24	14

Low-Fat Ice Cream with Poached Currants and Apples in Honey

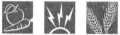

SERVES 4
35 MINUTES

1 medium Fuji or Granny Smith apple,
    peeled, cored, and cut into 8 pieces
½ cup water
¼ cup packed brown sugar
¼ cup currants
2 tablespoons honey
½ teaspoon cinnamon
4 scoops low-fat vanilla ice cream (3 ounces each)
1 tablespoon unsalted butter
1 teaspoon freshly squeezed lemon juice
Fresh basil

1   Place a 2-quart saucepan over medium heat.

2   Place all the ingredients in the pot except the ice cream, butter, lemon juice, and basil, and let simmer, stirring occasionally, until the sauce thickens, about 12–15 minutes.

3   When the sauce thickens, add the butter and the lemon and remove from the heat.

4   Place the scoops of ice cream in 4 serving bowls.

5   Pour the apple mixture over the ice cream and top each serving with a basil leaf.

Nutrient	Calories (kcal)	Carbohydrates (g)	Protein (g)	Fat (g)	Total Dietary Fiber (g)
Single Serving	272	56	3	4	7

Stir-Fry of Thin Steak, Garlic, Leek, Carrot, and Soy Ramen Noodles

SERVES 4
25 MINUTES

2 teaspoons toasted sesame oil

1 tablespoon canola oil

1 pound lean beef sirloin, trimmed of all fat and sliced into thin strips

1 medium leek, root end and 1 inch of green tips removed,
   outer layer discarded, sliced into ⅛-inch rounds

1 medium carrot, very thinly sliced

1 medium red bell pepper, cored, seeded, and cut into ⅛-inch strips

1 medium yellow bell pepper, cored, seeded, and cut into ⅛-inch strips

4 tablespoons low-sodium soy sauce

2 tablespoons freshly squeezed lemon juice

Salt to taste

QUICK NOODLES:

6 ounces ramen noodles,
   unseasoned

1 teaspoon kosher salt

1 teaspoon toasted sesame oil

1 Place a 3-quart saucepan filled ⅔ with water over high heat, add 1 teaspoon salt, and bring to a boil.

2 Add the noodles to the boiling water and turn down to a simmer for 3 minutes. Test the noodles by removing one, letting it cool, and tasting for texture.

3 Place a large sauté pan over high heat, add the sesame and canola oils, and heat about 1 minute—don't let it smoke.

4 | Add the beef, leek, carrot, and bell peppers to the sauté pan and cook for 5 minutes, stirring constantly.

5 | Turn the heat down to medium and add the soy sauce and lemon juice.

6 | Drain the cooked noodles, toss with the toasted sesame oil, and add to the beef and vegetables. Stir quickly and season with salt as needed.

Nutrient	Calories (kcal)	Carbohydrates (g)	Protein (g)	Fat (g)
Single Serving	441	42	30	17

Frozen Date and Pecan Yogurt

  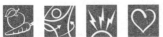

SERVES 4
20 MINUTES TO PREPARE, 2 HOURS FREEZING TIME

3 cups plain nonfat yogurt

¾ cup chopped dates

½ cup chopped pecans

⅓ cup honey

1 teaspoon ground coriander

½ teaspoon ground cinnamon

1 Place all the ingredients in a food processor and process until smooth.

2 Pour the mixture into a mixing bowl, cover, and freeze for 2 hours.

3 Just before serving, remove the yogurt from the freezer to soften, 4–5 minutes.

Nutrient	Calories (kcal)	Carbohydrates (g)	Protein (g)	Fat (g)
Single Serving	411	65	13	11

Slow-Cooked Garlic and Green Onion Vegetarian Stew

SERVES 4
2½ HOURS

2 small onions, thinly sliced

6 garlic cloves, roughly chopped

8 green onions (white part only), thinly sliced

1 medium leek (white part only), thinly sliced

1 stalk celery, finely diced

2 large tomatoes, cut into 8 pieces

1 large portobello mushroom cap, brushed clean with a dry towel
   and roughly chopped

1 large carrot, thinly sliced

1 sprig fresh thyme, or ½ teaspoon dried thyme

1 large russet potato, scrubbed and cut into 8 pieces

1 tablespoon molasses

4 cups water

Salt and pepper to taste

GARNISH:

¼ cup chopped parsley

1 tablespoon freshly squeezed lemon juice

2 tablespoons olive oil

Pinch salt

Pinch pepper

1 Place all the ingredients except the garnish in a Dutch oven. Bring to a boil, then reduce heat. Simmer for 2–2½ hours.

2 Just before serving, prepare the ingredients for the garnish, mix together, and stir into the pot.

Nutrient	Calories (kcal)	Carbohydrates (g)	Protein (g)	Fat (g)
Single Serving	117	23	4	1

3

KEY FOODS AND RECIPES FOR THE PREPARATION PERIOD

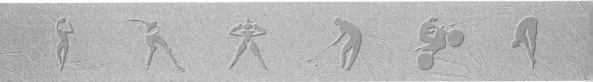

THE PREPARATION PERIOD FOLLOWS THE FOUNDATION PERIOD AND BUILDS upon the gains you've made in aerobic conditioning and strength. During this period, the intensity of your workouts increases, your training volume is pretty high, and your workouts are more sport-specific than they were in the Foundation Period. The aerobic and strength work from the Foundation Period improved your aerobic engine's capacity and the amount of total work you could do. The Preparation Period is the portion of the year when you more directly apply your increased capacity to your specific sport or activity.

Progression is one of the principles of training, meaning that in order for fitness and performance to continue improving, training has to progress so it still supplies sufficient stimulus for adaptation. With limited time available to train, many working adults have to increase the intensity of their workouts, rather than work out longer, in order to continue making progress in the Preparation Period. By doing so, you continue to develop your aerobic engine, but you're working at the upper limit of its capacity, so you're also calling upon the anaerobic system for some energy as well. Exercising at this harder, but sustainable, workload burns more calories per minute than your typical workouts in the Foundation Period, and a higher percentage of those calories are coming from carbohydrate.

The Preparation Period typically lasts 2–3 months or 3–4 macrocycles. For people living in the Northern Hemisphere and participating in primarily summer sports, this period usually occupies the late winter and spring (March–May, give or take a month or two). For folks who want to be in the best shape for winter sports, the Preparation Period would occupy summer and early fall months (September–November, give or take a month or two).

Feeding the Preparation Period

Since the volume of training is still pretty high and your intensity of training continues to build on the Foundation Period, your total caloric expenditure (and consequently your caloric demand) also increases as you enter the Preparation Period. The higher intensity causes an increase in carbohydrate usage, especially since your harder workouts call for a higher energy contribution from the anaerobic energy system. Your protein requirement also increases, since harder workouts cause more stress to muscles and your immune system. This increase in protein intake does not take much, if any, effort. For many active people, it's achieved in the process of consuming more calories.

In response to the increase in exercise intensity in the Preparation Period, you should increase your total caloric intake by about 15 percent. When described as a percentage increase, 15 percent is sometimes perceived as a license to heap more food on your plate, but in reality it only has small effects on portion sizes. For most people, increasing carbohydrate intake from the Foundation Period to the Preparation Period is only an addition of 60–90 grams per day. Spread across four to five meals and other snacks, this represents small increases (15–20 grams, less than one ounce) during each meal or snack.

For many people who are most active in the summer months, the Preparation Period falls in the spring months. This is often also the time when people seek to lose weight they gained during the previous cold months of winter. The caloric restriction necessary for weight loss is sometimes contradictory to your goal of improving fitness, especially when you have fewer than ten pounds to lose. Consuming too few calories to support your activity level results in poor training sessions, which in turn do not provide the stimulus necessary to lead to improvement. Perhaps more detrimental than poor training sessions is the struggle to recover from workouts that is also associated with a low energy intake. The

Transition and Foundation periods are better times of year to focus on weight loss, but if you find yourself with a few pounds to lose in the Preparation Period, be careful to limit your caloric deficit to about 500 calories per day.

Key Preparation Period Foods

In identifying key foods for the Preparation Period, I looked for concentrated sources of calories and carbohydrate so you can obtain the period's necessary energy increase through the addition of these ingredients to a wide variety of meals. Berries, as well as nuts and seeds, rarely make up a high proportion of an active person's caloric intake, but they can be a simple and healthy way to increase caloric intake without making major changes to the way you eat.

I selected whole-grain cereals as a key food group for the Preparation Period because they provide a lot of carbohydrate energy you need to prepare for your workouts and recover from them. While you can certainly eat whole-grain cereals by the bowlful, we incorporated them into different types of recipes in order to encourage increased variety in your food choices. Eating the same bowl of the same brand of cereal every morning for ten years is a better idea than eating doughnuts every morning, but the best option is to regularly change the type of cereal and the fruit on top. Variety is important in a nutrition program because it increases the sources from which you obtain different combinations of vitamins, minerals, phytochemicals, and flavonoids. The nutrients cereals, berries, and nuts and seeds bring in addition to their calories is a major reason for their inclusion in the Preparation Period.

Whole-Grain Cereals

Whole grains should be a staple of an active person's nutrition program, and they're not difficult to find. The grocery store shelves are packed with an ever-increasing number of whole-grain cereal products, from cereals to snack bars to breads. While many of these are ready-to-eat products, you can also integrate whole-grain cereals into recipes. Whole-grain cereals are those that contain the cracked, shelled, ground, or puffed kernel of grains like wheat, corn, or rice. The shell or husk of the kernel is important because it contains the majority of the micronutrients (vitamins, minerals, etc.) and fiber available in the food. Grains that have been processed to remove the husk deliver fewer micronutrients, have to be fortified, and are usually lower in fiber.

Fiber is an important component of whole-grain cereals because it has been shown to reduce your risk of developing cardiovascular disease and certain cancers. It also slows the digestion and absorption of carbohydrate energy, which can be both good and bad. When you need energy quickly, as from a preworkout snack, high-fiber foods may not be your best choice. On the other hand, high-fiber carbohydrate sources provide lasting energy, which make them ideal for inclusion into meals. The National Cancer Institute recommends a daily fiber intake of 25–30 grams, and whole-grain cereals are a great way to obtain a portion of this requirement.

Nuts and Seeds

Nuts and seeds contain carbohydrate, but it is their protein, unsaturated fatty acid, and antioxidant content that makes them a key food for the Preparation Period. While nuts and seeds do not contain complete protein, they are a good source of both essential and nonessential amino acids. Combining the protein, carbohydrate, and heart-healthy unsaturated fats, nuts and seeds pack a lot of energy into a small package. Adding nuts and seeds, or their oils, to recipes is a great way to increase the caloric content of a recipe while also increasing micronutrient and antioxidant intake.

Flaxseeds, flaxseed oil, sunflower seeds, almonds, cashews, peanuts, and peanut butter are good sources of vitamins E and A. Both of these vitamins have been shown to have significant antioxidant properties. They also deliver minerals, including selenium, magnesium, folate, and niacin. Peanuts are technically legumes, but they are commonly included with, and nutritionally resemble, nuts.

Flaxseed oil is also beneficial for your health. Like most vegetable oils, flaxseed oil contains linoleic acid, an essential fatty acid needed for survival. But unlike most oils, it also contains significant amounts of another essential fatty acid, alpha-linolenic acid (ALA). ALA converts in the body to the same heart-protective omega-3 fatty acids found in salmon, sardines, and mackerel. Although it is not suitable for cooking, flaxseed oil can be used in salads. You can also add flaxseed oil to a stir-fry or a pasta sauce, but you should stir it in right before serving. One tablespoon (15 ml) of flaxseed oil per day is recommended as a supplement in salad dressings or on vegetables to ensure a supply of essential fatty acids.

In comparison to flaxseed oil, it is less expensive to get your omega-3 fatty acids from the actual flaxseed. Flaxseeds are sold whole or ground, but they should be ground before use so they can be digested more readily. You don't need any special equipment for this process either; just throw whole flaxseeds in your coffee grinder. An ancient, but effective, mortar and pestle works well, too. In addition to sprinkling them on cereals, salads, casseroles, and desserts, ground flaxseeds can be used in baking to boost the nutritional content of cookies and brownies. Cooking does not significantly reduce the nutritional value of ground flaxseed, whereas flaxseed oil loses it beneficial properties if it's exposed to too much heat.

Berries

It's hard to imagine a world without berries. Strawberries, blueberries, blackberries, and raspberries are a tasty and nutrient-dense way to add a burst of flavor to any meal or snack. In terms of energy, they are a highly concentrated source of carbohydrate. One cup of blueberries, for instance, contains 21 grams of carbohydrate. Yet the most important contributions berries make to an active person's nutrition program come from the high concentrations of vitamin C, vitamin K, dietary fiber, antioxidants, and minerals they contain.

As with the other key Preparation Period foods, berries are a good way to add some carbohydrate energy to meals and snacks. All three of this period's key foods can be part of a single meal, like a bowl of oatmeal that has blueberries and almonds mixed in. Of course, as you'll see in the following pages, Mark Tarbell came up with more innovative ways to integrate these foods into your Preparation Period nutrition program.

Fresh Pear and Pecan Salad

SERVES 4
20 MINUTES

DRESSING:

2 tablespoons red wine vinegar

¼ cup olive oil

½ teaspoon brown sugar

½ teaspoon salt

Freshly ground black pepper

SALAD:

2 medium fresh Asian or Bartlett pears,
    cored and sliced into 10 pieces, skin left on

5 ounces baby frisée or baby escarole

5 ounces baby spinach

4 fresh dates, pitted and sliced into thin strips

¼ cup basil, hand torn

¼ cup Italian parsley, stemmed

1 green onion, thinly sliced

¼ cup crumbled blue cheese

¼ cup pecans, toasted (see Note)

1   In a small bowl, mix the red wine vinegar, olive oil, brown sugar, ½ teaspoon salt, and 2 twists of fresh pepper. Whisk for 30 seconds; set aside.

2   In a medium bowl, place the pears, frisée, spinach, dates, basil, parsley, and green onion. Toss lightly.

3   Add the dressing and toss together lightly.

4 | Divide evenly among 4 salad plates.

5 | Sprinkle with the blue cheese and pecan pieces.

NOTE: To toast pecan pieces, heat a nonstick pan over medium heat, add the pecans, and stir continuously for 5 minutes. Watch carefully to avoid burning. Remove from heat and let cool before using.

Nutrient	Calories (kcal)	Carbohydrates (g)	Protein (g)	Fat (g)
Single Serving	253	12	4	21

Good Basic Salad Dressing

MAKES ABOUT ¾ CUP; 2 TABLESPOONS PER SERVING
5 MINUTES

½ cup olive oil

3 tablespoons balsamic vinegar

1 tablespoon maple syrup

Salt to taste

In a small bowl, combine the olive oil, balsamic vinegar, maple syrup, and salt to taste.

Use for any salad greens or to brush over cooked meats, fish, or tofu. When using on lettuce the dressing should be a little salty as lettuce absorbs the flavor of salt.

Nutrient	Calories (kcal)	Carbohydrates (g)	Protein (g)	Fat (g)
Single Serving	174	3	0	18

Apricot–Toasted Almond Yogurt

SERVES 4
15 MINUTES

2 cups plain nonfat yogurt

4 tablespoons ground almonds

4 tablespoons apricot fruit-only spread/jam

⅛ teaspoon ground cinnamon

⅛ teaspoon salt

¼ cup sliced almonds, toasted

1 Place all ingredients except for the toasted almonds in a blender or food processor, and pulse the blender until smooth and well blended.

2 Serve in bowls with the toasted almonds sprinkled on top.

NOTE: To toast almonds, place a large nonstick skillet over medium-low to medium
heat. Add the sliced almonds and stir until just starting to turn golden brown.

Nutrient	Calories (kcal)	Carbohydrates (g)	Protein (g)	Fat (g)
Single Serving	194	25	10	6

Hearty Chicken Soup with Spinach and Rice

SERVES 4
30–40 MINUTES

4 cups organic or salt-free chicken broth

1 small onion, sliced

1 large organic tomato, cut into 8 pieces

4 tablespoons uncooked brown rice

2 cups tightly packed baby spinach

1 teaspoon low-sodium soy sauce

4 sprigs Italian parsley (leaves only)

Salt and pepper to taste

1 Place a 3- to 4-quart saucepan over medium to medium-high heat.

2 Add the chicken broth, sliced onion, tomato, and rice.

3 Bring to a low boil for 20 minutes.

4 Add the spinach, soy sauce, and parsley. Leave on low boil for 5 minutes.

5 Season with salt and pepper.

Nutrient	Calories (kcal)	Carbohydrates (g)	Protein (g)	Fat (g)
Single Serving	123	15	9	3

Broccoli Salad with Currants, Walnuts, and Blue Cheese

SERVES 4
10–25 MINUTES

SALAD:

2 heads fresh broccoli, cut into florets

¾ cup currants

½ cup coarsely chopped walnuts

½ cup crumbled blue cheese

2 tablespoons grated Parmesan cheese

DRESSING:

¾ cup nonfat sour cream

2 tablespoons freshly squeezed lemon juice

1 tablespoon honey

1 Optional: To steam broccoli: Place a 4-quart saucepan over high heat, fill ⅔ with water, bring to a boil, add pinch of salt, add broccoli florets, turn down to a low boil for 11 minutes, remove from heat, drain, and let cool.

2 Toss the broccoli, currants, and walnuts together in a large mixing bowl.

3 Stir all the dressing ingredients together in a medium mixing bowl until smooth.

4 Add the dressing to the broccoli mix.

5 Place the salad in a shallow bowl and sprinkle with the blue cheese and Parmesan.

Nutrient	Calories (kcal)	Carbohydrates (g)	Protein (g)	Fat (g)	Total Dietary Fiber (g)
Single Serving	354	48	18	10	11

Quick Whole-Wheat Biscuits

MAKES 12 BISCUITS
25 MINUTES

½ stick unsalted butter, cut into ½-inch cubes

1½ cups organic unbleached flour

¼ cup organic whole-wheat flour

¼ cup oat bran

4½ teaspoons baking powder

1 teaspoon sea salt

1 tablespoon sugar

⅔ cup heavy cream

1 Preheat the oven to 425°F.

2 Melt the butter in a saucepan and set aside.

3 Place all the dry ingredients, except 2 tablespoons of flour, in a food processor; pulse 5 times.

4 Add the cream and pulse until just starting to incorporate.

5 Turn out onto a cutting board and add the rest of the flour gently, just enough for the dough to come together.

6 On a lightly floured surface, roll dough out to a ¾-inch thickness. Cut with a 2- or 3-inch biscuit cutter.

7 Dip in the melted butter and place on a baking sheet.

8 Bake uncovered for 11–15 minutes, or until the tops are puffed up and light tan in color.

9 Serve warm, plain or with butter or honey.

Nutrient	Calories (kcal)	Carbohydrates (g)	Protein (g)	Fat (g)
Single Serving	157	16	3	9

Oat Bran, Currant, and Maple Muffins

  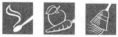

MAKES 24 MUFFINS
30 MINUTES

1 cup oat bran

1 cup unbleached all-purpose flour

1 tablespoon fresh baking powder*

1 teaspoon salt

1 cup currants

1½ cups 2 percent milk

⅓ cup maple syrup

3 tablespoons canola oil

1 large egg

1 | Preheat the oven to 400°F.

2 | In a large mixing bowl, combine the oat bran, flour, baking powder, and salt.

3 | In another mixing bowl, combine the currants, milk, maple syrup, canola oil, and egg.

4 | Combine all the ingredients and stir gently; there can be lumps in the mix.

5 | Grease a muffin tin and fill to ¾ from the top.

6 | Bake for 15–20 minutes.

NOTE: These muffins can be refrigerated and/or frozen in a tightly sealed container.

*Baking powder loses its effectiveness over time.

Nutrient	Calories (kcal)	Carbohydrates (g)	Protein (g)	Fat (g)
Single Serving	79	11	2	3

Oat Bran Super Drink with Almond Butter, Yogurt, and Blueberries

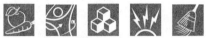

MAKES FOUR 14-OUNCE SERVINGS
20 MINUTES

2½ cups 1 percent milk

2½ cups plain nonfat yogurt

1 cup ripe blueberries, or ¾ cup frozen

4 tablespoons oat bran

3 tablespoons almond butter

5 tablespoons apricot fruit-only spread/jam

3 tablespoons honey

¼ teaspoon salt

1 Place all the ingredients in a blender.

2 Purée until smooth.

Nutrient	Calories (kcal)	Carbohydrates (g)	Protein (g)	Fat (g)
Single Serving	363	59	16	7

Quick Muesli with Apples and Oats

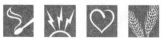

SERVES 4
30 MINUTES

3 cups rolled oats

2 medium apples (your favorite), grated or shredded

½ cup chopped almonds

¾ cup currants or raisins

1 tablespoon bee pollen (optional, check if allergic)

1 tablespoon unsalted, shelled sunflower seeds

¼ cup chopped dried apricots or fresh grapes

¾ cup warm water

4 tablespoons honey

OPTIONAL:

Substitute apple juice for water.

Add ¼ teaspoon cinnamon.

1 | Stir together all the ingredients except the warm water and honey in a large mixing bowl.

2 | Stir in the warm water and honey. (You can add more or less water to make the desired consistency.)

Nutrient*	Calories (kcal)	Carbohydrates (g)	Protein (g)	Fat (g)
Single Serving	699	118	23	15

*Optional ingredients not included in these numbers.

Whole-Wheat Tuna Melt with Currants and Dill

  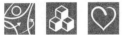

SERVES 4
25 MINUTES

2 cans (6 ounces each) white tuna, drained

¼ cup canned chickpeas (garbanzo beans), drained

¼ medium yellow onion, finely diced

1 stalk celery, diced

¾ cup low-fat sour cream

3 teaspoons chopped fresh dill, or 1 teaspoon dried dillweed

1 teaspoon salt

1 teaspoon black pepper

1 tablespoon grated Parmesan cheese

4 slices whole-wheat bread, toasted dry (no butter)

¾ cup grated Monterey Jack cheese for melting on top

1 Preheat the broiler on low or medium setting, or place under the broiler one shelf down from the top.

2 Mix all the ingredients except the whole-wheat toast and the grated Monterey Jack cheese in a large bowl.

3 Place the toast on a baking sheet and divide the tuna mixture evenly.

4 Spread the Monterey Jack cheese evenly on the top of each serving.

5 Place under the broiler until the cheese is fully melted, removing just before it browns.

NOTE: You can make the tuna mixture ahead of time; remove it from refrigerator 15 minutes prior to assembly.

Nutrient	Calories (kcal)	Carbohydrates (g)	Protein (g)	Fat (g)
Single Serving	356	21	32	16

Chicken Tortilla Soup

SERVES 4
1 HOUR

12 ounces boneless, skinless chicken breast,
    cut into ½-inch strips
    (Vegan: Substitute 10 ounces fresh tofu,
    2 tablespoons soy miso,
    and 2 tablespoons low-sodium soy sauce.)
4 cups chicken broth
    (Vegan: Substitute 4 cups vegetable broth.)
2 cups water
2 medium tomatoes,
    cored and chopped into ½-inch pieces
1 medium yellow onion,
    coarsely chopped
3 garlic cloves, chopped into ¼-inch pieces
1 large poblano chili pepper, cored, seeded,
    and cut into ½-inch pieces
3 small corn tortillas, ripped into 2-inch pieces
2 tablespoons red chili powder
1 teaspoon ground cumin
2 tablespoons white vinegar
2 tablespoons freshly squeezed lime juice
½ bunch cilantro, leaves only
Salt and pepper to taste

1 Place all the ingredients except for lime juice, cilantro, salt, and pepper in a 4-quart saucepan over high heat until boiling.

2 Turn the heat down to a low boil and cook for 25 minutes.

3 | Turn heat down to a simmer for 10 minutes. It can be served right away or may simmer for up to 30 more minutes.

4 | Just before serving, stir in lime juice, cilantro, salt, and pepper.

Nutrient	Calories (kcal)	Carbohydrates (g)	Protein (g)	Fat (g)
Single Serving	179	16	22	3

Spicy Three-Egg Arizona Scramble

SERVES 1
30 MINUTES

2 tablespoons canola oil

¼ medium yellow onion, roughly chopped

½ large poblano chili pepper, cored, seeded, and cut into ½-inch pieces

1 small red or green jalapeño pepper, cored, seeded,
    and chopped into ⅛-inch pieces

1 teaspoon red chili powder

1 teaspoon ground cumin

3 large eggs, beaten

½ medium tomato, cored and chopped into ½-inch pieces

2 teaspoon white vinegar

Salt and pepper to taste

2 tablespoons cilantro, leaves only

1 tablespoon low-fat sour cream

Freshly squeezed lime juice

Tabasco sauce (optional)

1 | Place a large sauté pan over medium-high heat and, when hot, add the canola oil.

2 | Add the onions, peppers, and spices and cook, stirring, for 3 minutes.

3 | In a large mixing bowl, beat the eggs, tomato, vinegar, and salt and pepper. Add to the pan, lower heat, and stir until the eggs are cooked.

4 | Toss the eggs on a plate and garnish with cilantro, sour cream, lime juice, and hot sauce, if desired.

Nutrient	Calories (kcal)	Carbohydrates (g)	Protein (g)	Fat (g)
Single Serving	255	21	18	11

Whole-Wheat Spaghetti with
Toasted Pumpkin Seeds and Cilantro

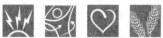

SERVES 4
25 MINUTES

SAUCE:

⅔ cup olive oil

3 tablespoons water

2 tablespoons freshly squeezed lemon juice

¼ cup pumpkin seeds, toasted in a dry sauté pan for 3 minutes

¼ cup pine nuts

3 leaves basil

½ bunch cilantro, stemmed, reserving several leaves for garnish

¼ small jalepeño pepper, seeded and finely minced
    (Note: After handling peppers, be careful not to touch
    sensitive areas of skin on your body;
    juice from the peppers can cause burning and discomfort.)

2 tablespoons grated Parmesan cheese and 2 tablespoons
    for sprinkling on top

1 teaspoon ground cumin

Salt and pepper to taste

PASTA:

1 teaspoon salt

8 ounces whole-wheat spaghetti

1 tablespoon olive oil

1 Place all the sauce ingredients in a blender and process on high until smooth. You may have to add more water to loosen up the sauce.

2 Place a 3-quart saucepan filled ⅔ with water over high heat and add the 1 teaspoon of salt.

3 | When boiling, add the pasta, stir, and reduce heat to a low boil for about 6 minutes, until al dente.

4 | Pull a piece of pasta out, set on a plate, and let cool a minute. Taste for doneness.

5 | Drain the pasta and toss in the olive oil.

6 | While still warm toss with the sauce, top with the cilantro, and serve immediately.

Nutrient	Calories (kcal)	Carbohydrates (g)	Protein (g)	Fat (g)
Single Serving	748	51	19	52

Yogurt with Toasted Pecans and Maple Syrup

 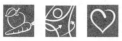

SERVES 4
20 MINUTES

6 ounces pecans, finely chopped

1 pint (16 ounces) plain nonfat yogurt

¼ cup and 1 tablespoon maple syrup

¼ teaspoon cinnamon

4 medium strawberries, hulled

1 Place a nonstick skillet over medium heat, add pecans, and stir for 3 minutes. Remove and set aside to cool.

2 Place all the ingredients except the strawberries in a medium mixing bowl and stir until blended.

3 Serve in bowls with a strawberry on top of each serving.

Nutrient	Calories (kcal)	Carbohydrates (g)	Protein (g)	Fat (g)
Single Serving	451	33	10	31

Black Raspberry and Candied-Walnut Yogurt

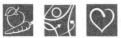

SERVES 4
20 MINUTES

⅔ cup walnuts, finely chopped

1 tablespoon water

3 tablespoons brown sugar

1 tablespoon unsalted butter

¼ teaspoon salt

1 pint (16 ounces) plain nonfat yogurt

¼ cup and 1 tablespoon black raspberry fruit-only spread/jam

¼ teaspoon ground coriander

4 mint sprigs

1 | Place a nonstick pan over medium heat.

2 | Add the walnuts, 1 tablespoon water, and sugar to the pan and stir until the sugar melts and starts bubbling.

3 | When the sugar is browning, add the butter and salt and stir until the butter has melted.

4 | Remove the mixture from the pan and set aside to cool.

5 | Place all the ingredients except the mint in a medium mixing bowl and stir until blended.

6 | Serve in bowls with a mint sprig on top of each serving.

Nutrient	Calories (kcal)	Carbohydrates (g)	Protein (g)	Fat (g)
Single Serving	324	36	9	16

Fresh Blueberry Pudding with Brown-Sugar Yogurt

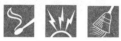

SERVES 4
20 MINUTES

1 pint fresh blueberries

¼ cup honey

¼ teaspoon cinnamon

1 pint (16 ounces) plain nonfat yogurt

3 tablespoons brown sugar

4 mint sprigs

1 Place the blueberries, honey, and cinnamon in food processor and process until smooth.

2 Put the blueberry mixture in 4 separate bowls and place in the refrigerator to chill.

3 Mix the yogurt and brown sugar together in a medium mixing bowl, stirring until blended.

4 Remove the blueberry mixture from the refrigerator.

5 Spoon the yogurt mixture over, dividing evenly.

6 Place a mint sprig on top of each serving.

Nutrient	Calories (kcal)	Carbohydrates (g)	Protein (g)	Fat (g)
Single Serving	224	51	5	0

Homemade Health Bar

MAKES ONE 4X7-INCH LOAF (12 SERVINGS)
20 MINUTES

1½ cups almonds

1 cup walnuts

½ cup pine nuts

½ cup raw, unsalted peanuts

1 cup rolled oats

1 cup oat bran

¼ cup flaxseed

1½ cups organic dates, chopped

1 cup organic currants

1 cup organic dried apricots, halved

½ cup organic dried apples, chopped

¼ cup organic raisins

1 tablespoon ground nutmeg

1 tablespoon ground cinnamon

1 teaspoon salt

Approximately ¾ cup spring water

1   Place all the ingredients except the water in a large mixing bowl and stir together.

2   Place a quarter at a time in a food processor and process until smooth, approximately 6 minutes.

3   Place all the chopped ingredients in a large mixing bowl, stir once more, and add the water until the mixture just comes together.

4.   Spread the mixture out on a cutting board, press together, and wrap or pack in plastic bags. Store in the refrigerator.

Nutrient	Calories (kcal)	Carbohydrates (g)	Protein (g)	Fat (g)	Total Dietary Fiber (g)
Single Serving	412	56	11	16	10

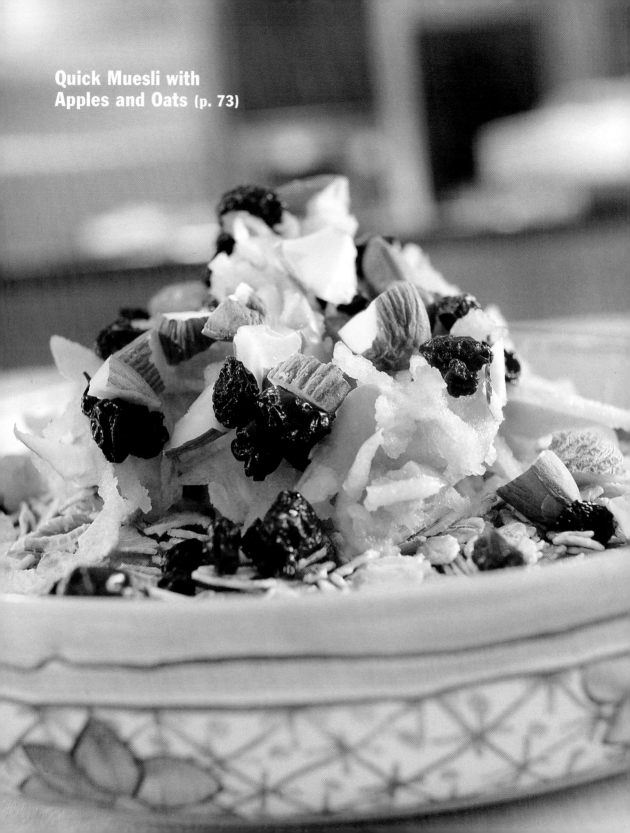

Quick Muesli with
Apples and Oats (p. 73)

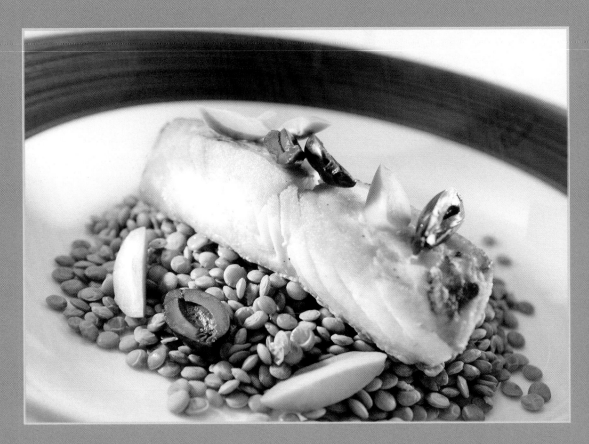

**Roasted Halibut with Mediterranean
Lentils and Olives** (p. 36)

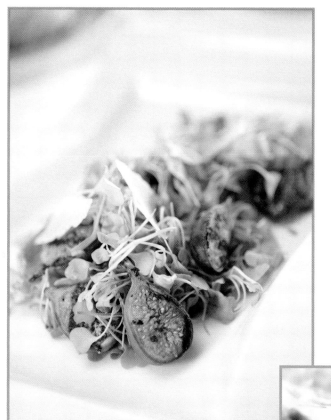

**Warm Fig and
Arugula Salad** (p. 32)

Oven-Roasted Garlic (p. 27)

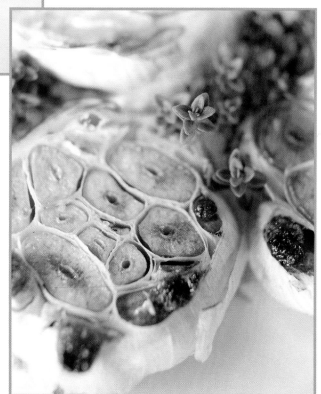

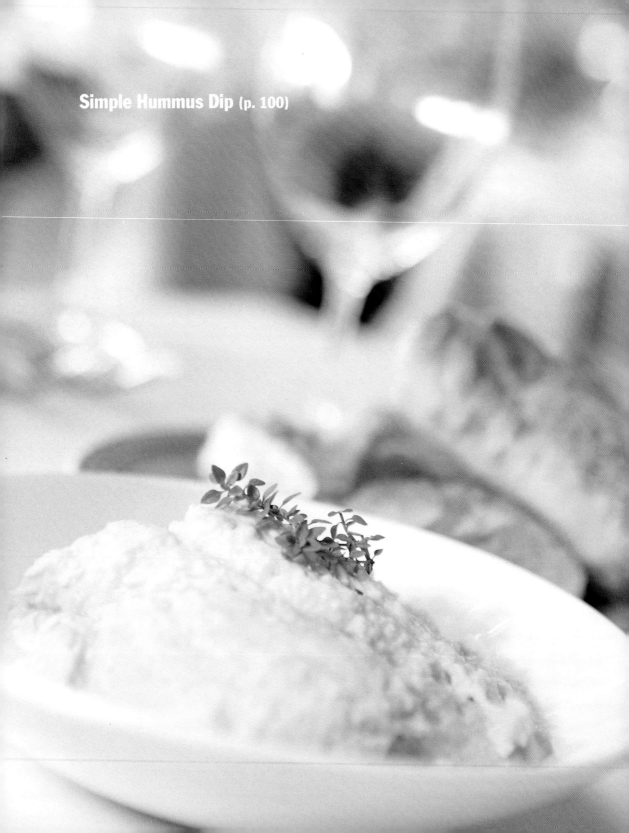
Simple Hummus Dip (p. 100)

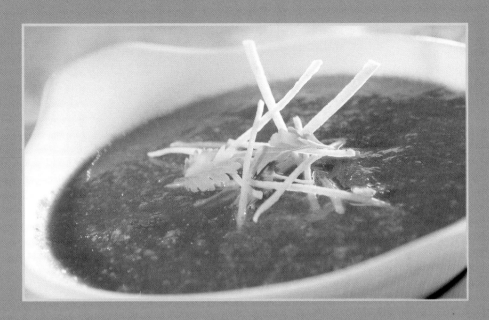

Chicken Tortilla Soup (p. 75)

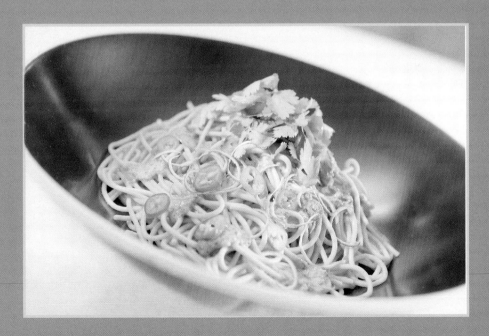

**Whole-Wheat Spaghetti
with Toasted Pumpkin Seeds and Cilantro** (p. 77)

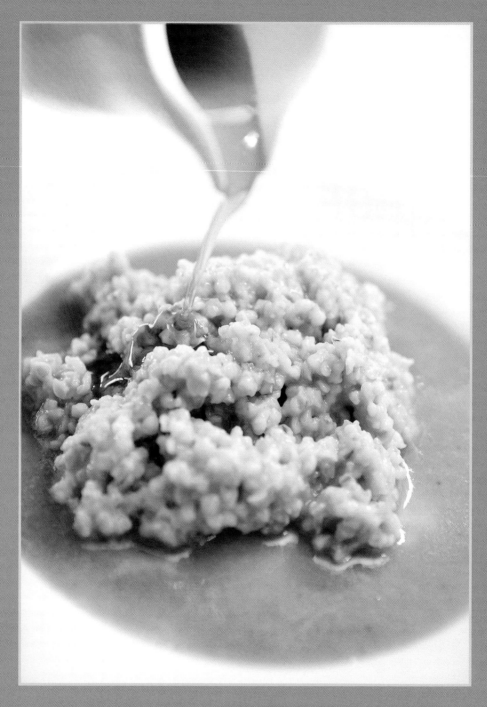

**Steel-Cut Oatmeal with Maple Syrup
and Strawberry Sauce (p. 83)**

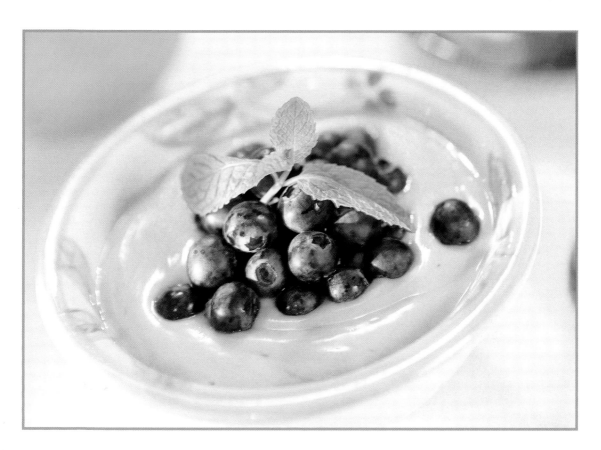

Fresh Blueberry Pudding with Brown-Sugar Yogurt (p. 81)

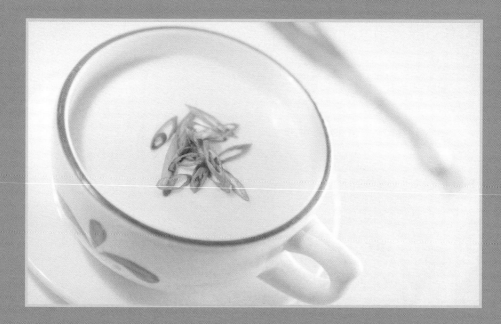

Russet Potato and Green Onion Soup (p. 115)

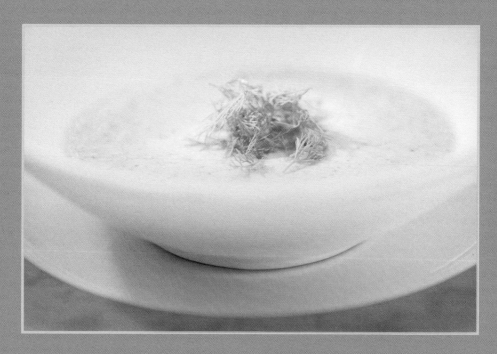

Creamy Soybean Soup (p. 101)

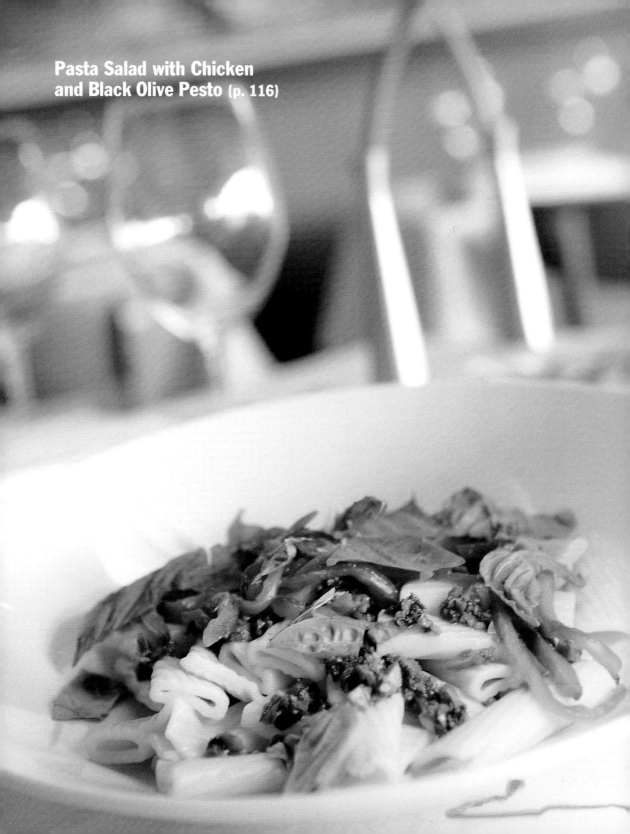

Pasta Salad with Chicken
and Black Olive Pesto (p. 116)

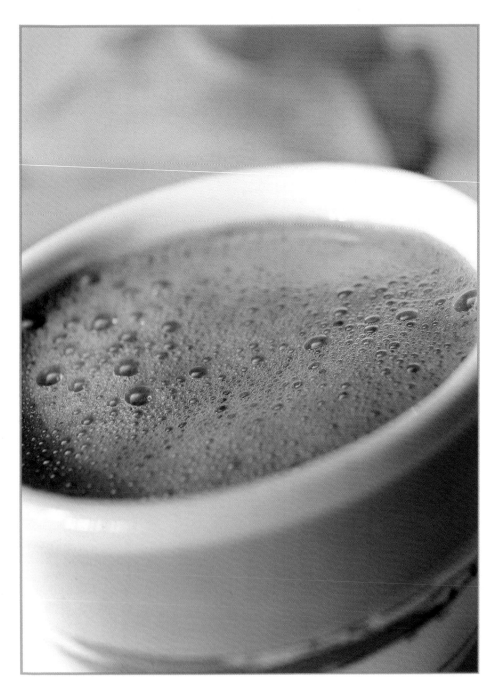

Chilled Watermelon Soup (p. 118)

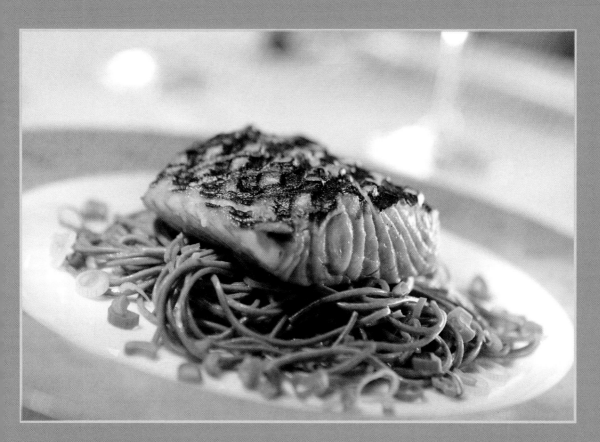

**Broiled Salmon on Buckwheat Noodles
with Ginger and Soy** (p. 108)

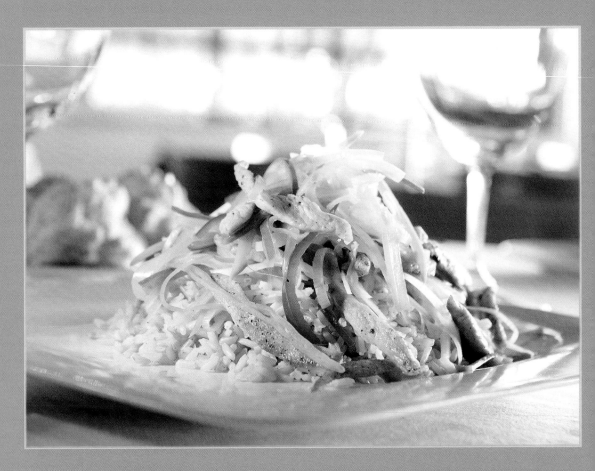

One-Pan Chicken and Legume Stir-Fry (p. 122)

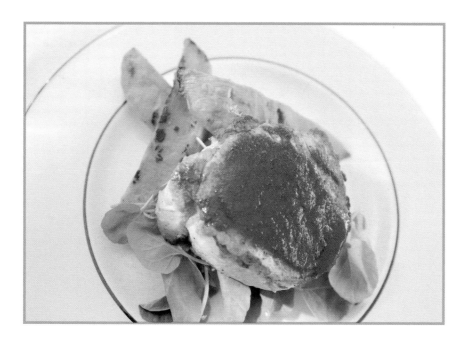

Red Chili and Honey Rubbed Pork Sirloin with Sweet Potato Spears (p. 110)

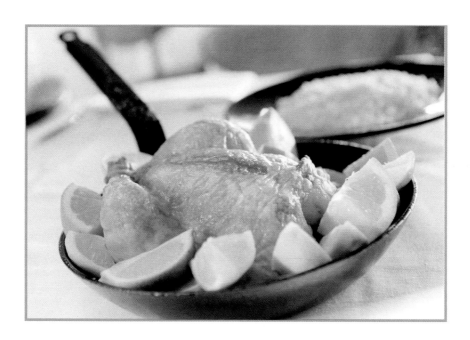

Roasted Citrus-Stuffed Chicken with Couscous (p. 125)

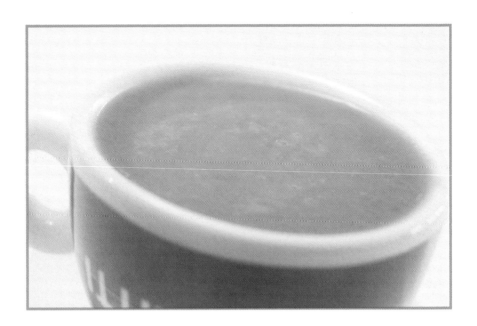

Red Lentil and Carrot Soup (p. 133)

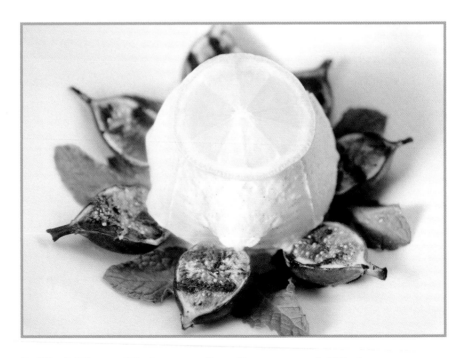

Grilled Figs with Lemon Ice Cream and Mint (p. 163)

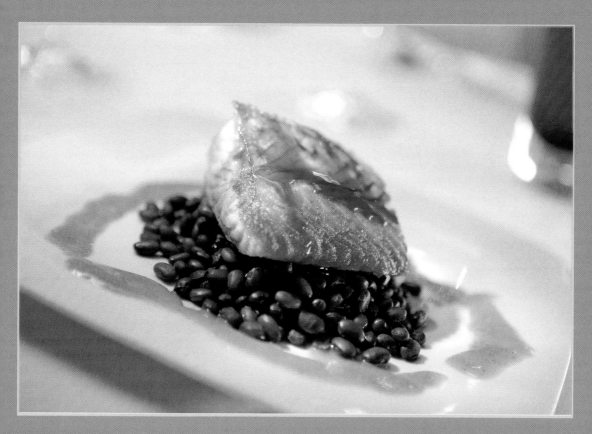

Ancho-Roasted Salmon with Black Beans and Kiwi Sauce (p. 156)

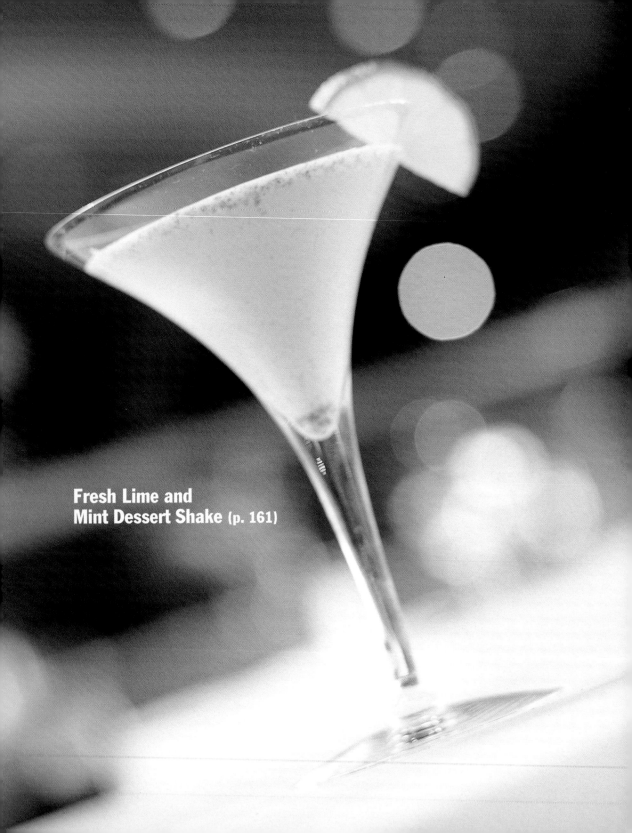

**Fresh Lime and
Mint Dessert Shake** (p. 161)

Steel-Cut Oatmeal with Maple Syrup and Strawberry Sauce

  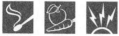

SERVES 4
45 MINUTES

5 cups water

1 cup steel-cut (not rolled) oats

½ cup maple syrup

¼ teaspoon cinnamon

Strawberry Sauce (page 84)

1 Place a 3-quart saucepan over high heat and add the water.

2 Bring the water to a boil and add the steel-cut oats.

3 Turn the heat down to a very slow simmer for 25–35 minutes, stirring occasionally. You must watch the heat and turn down more and more as the oatmeal begins to thicken.

4 Remove from the heat and stir in the maple syrup and cinnamon.

5 Serve with Strawberry Sauce, if desired.

Nutrients*	Calories (kcal)	Carbohydrates (g)	Protein (g)	Fat (g)
Single Serving	163	52	7	3

*Strawberry Sauce not included in these numbers.

Strawberry Sauce

MAKES ABOUT 3 CUPS (2 TABLESPOONS PER SERVING)
5 MINUTES

1 pint ripe strawberries, hulled and halved

2 tablespoons maple syrup

3 tablespoons strawberry fruit-only spread/jam

1 Place all the ingredients in a blender and process until smooth.

2 Pour the sauce over ice cream, yogurt, or warm oatmeal. Will keep, covered, in refrigerator for 3 days.

Nutrient	Calories (kcal)	Carbohydrates (g)	Protein (g)	Fat (g)
Single Serving	12	3	0	0

Lemon Feta Vinaigrette

MAKES ABOUT ¾ CUP (2 TABLESPOONS PER SERVING)
10 MINUTES

½ cup olive oil

1–2 tablespoons freshly squeezed lemon juice

⅓ cup crumbled Feta cheese

   (Vegan: Use soy provolone or cheddar cheese tossed in a small mixing bowl

   with 2 tablespoons white vinegar and 1 teaspoon salt.)

2 teaspoons finely chopped oregano (or ½ teaspoon dried)

Salt to taste

1 Mix the ingredients in a small mixing bowl, adding the lemon juice 1 tablespoon at a time to adjust for taste.

2 Spoon over grilled fish or tofu.

Nutrient	Calories (kcal)	Carbohydrates (g)	Protein (g)	Fat (g)
Single Serving	182	1	1	20

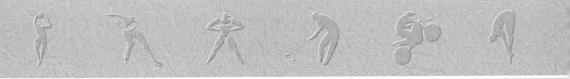

KEY FOODS AND RECIPES FOR
THE SPECIALIZATION PERIOD

EVEN IF YOU HAVE NO DESIRE TO COMPETE, THERE IS MOST LIKELY A POR-
tion of the year when you would like to be in your best shape. Some active people don't necessarily train for specific events, but rather aim to be in top condition to participate in a
variety of activities in a given season. The summer-sport enthusiast, for instance, strives to
be in good shape as the season begins because outdoor activities are more fun when you are
physically prepared for them. Downhill skiers and snowboarders aim to be in top shape
when the snow starts falling because the ski season lasts only for a few months. They don't
want to waste half the season skiing half days and feeling tired before they get in shape. Being in optimal shape for your favorite season of the year gives you the opportunity to make
the most of that season while it lasts.

Competitive athletes build their periodization plans around being optimally prepared
for one event or a series of events. In Lance Armstrong's case, the Tour de France falls right
in the middle of his Specialization Period. The period begins about six weeks prior to the
beginning of July, the month when the three-week race is held. In these final weeks build-

ing up to the Tour, Lance's training is very intense, but the volume decreases. He spends fewer hours on the bike than during the Preparation Period, but his workouts are harder than at any other time of the year.

The training intensity in your Specialization Period needs to be very high, because this is the time of year when you are working on systems that supply energy for maximal efforts. At the same time, this is the most thrilling part of the year for many active people because this is when you are at the height of your fitness. The positive side of increased intensity is that the workouts are shorter, and your overall training volume decreases. The harder you work, the more recovery you need; and in the Specialization Period, you're either working at full throttle or you're resting. Failing to get enough rest during the Specialization Period will undermine your performance more than any other factor. With insufficient recovery, you won't be able to give your best efforts in training and you may jeopardize your chances of reaching your competitive goals or having the energy to participate fully in your preferred activities.

Body Weight in the Specialization Period

In Chapter 1, I talked about the mismatch between energy intake and energy expenditure that is common for active individuals who don't follow a periodized nutrition program. During certain portions of the year, these people consume more food than they need, and consequently gain weight. They then work harder or eat less during the Preparation Period to lose weight, because they want to reach the Specialization Period at their "fighting weight." They want to be lean and looking good for their goal event or most active time period. The trouble is, the typical nonperiodized nutrition program doesn't provide enough energy to support Specialization Period activities.

Refer to Figure 1 on page 5 for a minute. The curve that represents energy expenditure is much higher than the line for energy intake during the Specialization Period. This is significant for two reasons: you lose weight whenever energy out is greater than energy in; and both performance and your ability to recover suffer dramatically when you fail to consume enough energy to support your activities.

Any weight-loss goals you might have should be completed before you begin the Specialization Period. This is a time when energy is at a premium and you need every calorie you consume. At the elite level of sports, the demands are extreme and athletes go to extremes to prepare for competition. Lance Armstrong's Tour de France weight is not sustainable or healthy for more than a few weeks, but it's an important component to winning the race. For active people and amateur competitors, you're going to perform better, and feel better, as a result of eating copious amounts of nutrient-rich, calorie-dense foods during the Specialization Period. The positive impacts of quality training, adequate rest, and sufficient energy intake will outweigh (no pun intended) the potential effects of being a few pounds lighter.

By matching your nutrition program to your activity level throughout the year, your body weight will be relatively stable. You will naturally gain and lose a few pounds as activity level changes, but such fluctuations are normal and healthy. Instead of having to proactively lose a chunk of weight at once, your body weight will gradually decrease during the Preparation and Specialization periods, without the need to increase training or restrict food. All the while, consuming sufficient energy allows you to have quality workouts and optimal recovery, which in turn leads to greater performance.

Feeding the Specialization Period

Nutrition plays a major role in the success of your Specialization Period. High-intensity training, frequent hard exercise, and participation in goal events requires a lot of carbohydrate for fuel, and the workouts during this period will burn through your body's carbohydrate stores faster than any other portion of the year. The stress induced by these workouts also increases the importance of protein in your nutrition program, as there is a lot of muscle repair going on in the Specialization Period. The immune system takes a beating during this period as well. Ironically, as you get closer to performing at your absolute best, your risk of getting sick increases. After working so hard to be in top shape, don't let yourself be undermined by poor recovery and nutritional choices.

Carbohydrate is the most important nutrient for success in the Specialization Period. As you go from a walking pace to an all-out effort, the rate at which you burn carbohydrate increases fivefold. At this time of year, you're spending more time near the upper end of that scale than during any previous period. The more carbohydrate you burn during exercise, the more you need to consume beforehand to prepare, and afterward to recover.

The timing of your postworkout meal is very important all year, and especially critical during the Specialization Period. During the first 15–60 minutes after exercise, your muscles can take in carbohydrate and protein at their highest rates. Replenishing carbohydrate stores and speeding protein to muscle cells is a critical step in the recovery process. Numerous studies agree that having full carbohydrate stores at the beginning of exercise improves performance and prolongs time to exhaustion. Take advantage of your body's built-in recovery accelerator; consume a high-carbohydrate drink, snack, or meal within the first hour after exercise. Including some protein in this food may help accelerate the process, but since it won't lead to increased carbohydrate storage, be careful not to let the protein displace the calories you really need from carbohydrate.

With caloric intake at its highest level of the year, protein intake will also be highest during the Specialization Period. It is important to realize, however, that even at its highest level, protein intake is not terribly high. While active people and athletes require more protein than sedentary people, consuming more than about 0.9–1.0 gram of protein per pound of body weight per day doesn't provide additional benefits. In other words, there's no reason to oversupply your body with protein. High-quality, low-fat cuts of meat, fish, and poultry, as well as eggs and soy products, are among your best choices because they provide complete protein, a lot of vitamins, minerals, antioxidants, and phytochemicals in a relatively small number of calories. This leaves more room in your nutrition program for carbohydrate, the high-octane fuel necessary for speed, power, focus, and agility.

The Specialization Period is the only time of the year when you should pay a little more attention to your fat intake. You need a lot of energy during this period, and the fuel you're looking for is clean-burning carbohydrate. You also need an elevated protein intake for your muscles and immune system. When you're consuming so much food, it is easy to believe that any food you can get your hands on is all right to eat. Many athletes can meet their carbohydrate and protein needs, but they inadvertently pile on mountains of excess fat calories in the process. That being said, you shouldn't go to drastic measures to reduce fat intake. Rather than looking for ways to remove as much fat from your nutrition program as possible, try to minimize the amount of fat that gets added to your daily intake when you move into the Specialization Period. As a result, you'll achieve the majority of the caloric increase from carbohydrate, some from protein, and a smaller portion from fat.

Key Specialization Period Foods

The Specialization Period has long been the time when athletes forgo variety and instead shovel massive portions of the same high-energy foods down their throats for weeks on end. While that method is reasonably effective, it's boring, and a person can only thrive on spaghetti and baked potatoes for so long. The Specialization Period can be very taxing on the mind; you're working hard and you're often tired, and the pressure wears some people down faster than others. A stale nutrition program can hasten this process because you get tired of eating the same old starch every meal. While this period's key foods—whole grains, dark-colored vegetables, and poultry—are pretty much the staples of a high-energy diet, Mark Tarbell did a wonderful job of developing new ways to prepare them and keep things interesting.

Whole Grains

While I talked about whole-grain cereals in the Preparation Period, there's more to whole grains than cereal. In the Specialization Period, grains are going to be a component of almost every meal and snack you consume. That doesn't mean everything has to be whole-wheat bread or brown rice either; expand your horizons to try barley, quinoa, whole-grain corn, couscous, and rye.

In addition to a lot of carbohydrate energy, these grains are good sources of a variety of minerals, including iron, selenium, and manganese. Iron plays an important role in your ability to transport oxygen in the blood, and while many active people fulfill their iron requirements with a combination of animal and plant sources, vegetarians have to be careful about iron intake. The iron from plant sources is not as readily usable by the body, meaning vegetarians actually have higher iron requirements than meat eaters. The general recommendations for iron are 8 milligrams/day (mg/d) for men and 18 mg/d for women. For vegetarians, these increase to 14 mg/d for men and 33 mg/d for women. Vitamin C increases the absorption of iron for both meat eaters and vegetarians, making that glass of orange juice, handful of berries, tablespoon of jam, or side of colorful vegetables even more valuable than it already was.

Colorful Vegetables

While you can't tell anything about a person by the color of his or her skin, you can tell a lot from the color of a vegetable. Pale, white, and faintly colored vegetables tend to contain lower concentrations of vitamins, minerals, and antioxidants. Darker, brighter, and more vibrantly colored vegetables, on the other hand, are packed with beneficial nutrients. When you're looking for the biggest bang for your buck in vegetables, fill your basket with the richest, most lustrous colors you can find.

Generally speaking, the more vibrant and intense the color, the higher a fruit or vegetable's content of vitamins, minerals, antioxidants, and carotenoids. Carotenoids include beta-carotene, lutein, and lycopene, and evidence suggests these compounds found in colorful vegetables may help prevent degenerative eye diseases and some forms of cancer.

Dark green varieties of lettuce like romaine or mignonette, red and yellow peppers, spinach, broccoli, and sweet potatoes are all high-quality carriers. In contrast, vegetables that lack color often contain fewer beneficial components. Since they still contain some vitamins, minerals, antioxidants, and phytochemicals, they are still considered quality carriers, but they shouldn't be your first choice at the vegetable stand. Iceberg lettuce, cucumbers, celery, and white mushrooms are good additions to many recipes, but you shouldn't look to them as major sources of nutrition.

The following table lists a variety of vegetables, based on a nutrition score. The Center for Science in the Public Interest (CSPI) devised the scoring system by looking at the effectiveness of vegetables in delivering seven nutrients: carotenoids, vitamins C and K, folate,

Vegetable	Nutrient Score*	Nutrient Highlights	
		High in... (20–100+ % DV)	Moderate (10–19% DV) or adequate (5–9% DV) source of...
Sweet potato (baked w/skin)	424	Carotenoids, vitamins C	Potassium, fiber, folate
Spinach (raw)	287	Carotenoids, vitamin K	Folate, vitamin C
Red pepper	261	Carotenoids, very high in vitamin C	N/A
Butternut squash	176	Carotenoids, vitamin C	Fiber
Romaine lettuce	174	Carotenoids, vitamins C and K	Folate, potassium
Asparagus	163	Vitamin K, folate	Vitamin C, carotenoids, fiber
Baked potato w/skin	139	Vitamin C, iron, potassium, fiber	Folate
Green pepper	109	Vitamin C	Vitamin K
Frozen peas	104	Carotenoids, vitamin K	Fiber, vitamin C, folate, iron
Baked potato w/out skin	69	Vitamin C	Potassium, fiber
Corn	67	Carotenoids	Vitamin C, folate, potassium, fiber
Iceberg lettuce	45	Vitamin K	Carotenoids, folate
Onions	31	N/A	Vitamin C, fiber
Cucumber	14	N/A	N/A
Mushrooms (raw)	11	N/A	N/A

potassium, iron, and fiber. While you should consume more of the high-scoring vegetables, low-scoring vegetables aren't bad for you; they just don't provide as many nutrients. If you're preparing mixed vegetables or a salad, make sure you have a few high-scoring vegetables in there, and then throw in any other vegetables you like.

While all vegetables supply beneficial nutrients, not all of them are good sources of carbohydrate fuel. For instance, spinach is packed with nutrients that support your health and performance, but a cup of it supplies less than 6 grams of carbohydrate, four of which are fiber. This certainly doesn't mean you shouldn't eat spinach, but you have to realize it would take an enormous amount of spinach to fulfill a large portion of your daily carbohydrate energy needs. The same is true of the varieties of peppers and lettuces: great nutritional value, but low on fuel. The table below shows some of the best vegetable choices for nutrient density as well as energy:

Vegetable	Grams of Carbohydrate Per Cup
Baked potato w/skin	51
Sweet potato (baked w/skin)	48
Garbanzo beans	45
White or yellow corn, boiled	41
Butternut squash	21
Green peas, boiled	25

Poultry

Chicken and turkey are wonderful sources of complete protein, iron, zinc, and numerous vitamins year round. Since they are low in total fat and saturated fat, once you remove the skin, they are very well suited to the Specialization Period. Essentially, they are a relatively low-calorie source of high-quality protein, leaving more room in your nutrition program for carbohydrate calories.

While white meat, as in the breast, is the most commonly eaten portion of chicken and turkey, dark meat is also beneficial. Even though dark meat is higher in fat than white meat, it is also higher in zinc and iron. Dark meat contains twice as much iron as white meat and three times as much zinc. Zinc plays an important role in maintaining the immune system; and since the intensity of the Specialization Period exacts a heavy toll on the immune system, this is an important consideration at this time of year.

Seven-Layer Turkey Casserole with Brown Rice and Sweet Corn

SERVES 6
2 HOURS

1 cup uncooked brown rice

1 can (about 15 ounces) organic spring peas, drained,
     or 1½ cups frozen organic peas (do not defrost)

½ cup organic chicken broth

Dash salt and pepper

1½ cups chopped tomato

3 garlic cloves, finely chopped

½ onion, finely chopped

12 ounces ground turkey

Dash salt and pepper

½ cup chopped tomato

4 tablespoons organic chicken broth

2 cups fresh spinach, chopped into 1-inch pieces

1½ cups grated Monterey Jack cheese

1 Layer all ingredients from the brown rice through the spinach in the order listed in a 2- to 3-quart casserole.

2 Bake, covered, for 1 hour at 350°F.

3 Remove cover and spread the Monterey Jack cheese on top.

4 Bake uncovered for 30 more minutes.

Nutrient	Calories (kcal)	Carbohydrates (g)	Protein (g)	Fat (g)
Single Serving	254	33	17	6

Suzy's White Bean Chili

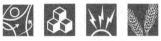

SERVES 4
1½ HOURS

6 cups organic free-range chicken stock

1½ pounds boneless, skinless chicken breast

2 tablespoons canola or olive oil

1 large yellow onion, roughly diced

1 can (16 ounces) white beans

1 large Anaheim pepper, seeded and roughly diced

2 tablespoons ground cumin

2 tablespoons ancho or regular chili powder

1 tablespoon freshly ground black pepper

1 tablespoon chopped oregano, or 1 teaspoon good-quality dried oregano

Kosher salt to taste

1 tablespoon chopped cilantro

1 | Bring the chicken stock to a strong simmer over medium or medium-high heat.

2 | Add the chicken breast and simmer for 17 minutes, or until there is no pink left in the middle.

3 | When fully cooked, remove the chicken and set aside to cool.

4 | Remove the chicken stock from heat and set aside.

5 | Place a 4-quart saucepan over medium heat for 1 minute and add the oil.

6 | Heat the oil for 1 minute, add the diced onion, and sauté for 5 minutes, stirring occasionally; do not let brown.

7 | Add the ground cumin and chili powder to the onion and stir over medium heat for 2 minutes.

8 | Add the reserved chicken stock and the remaining ingredients except the salt and cilantro.

9 Pull the chicken breast by hand into small pieces and add to saucepan.

10 Bring to a boil, then simmer for 30 minutes and season to taste with salt.

11 Just before serving, add chopped cilantro.

NOTE: It gets better if refrigerated for one day. Reheat the next day.

Nutrient	Calories (kcal)	Carbohydrates (g)	Protein (g)	Fat (g)
Single Serving	673	80	59	13

Sweet Potato and Garlic Soup

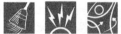

SERVES 4
1½ HOURS

3 tablespoons olive oil

1 medium onion, finely diced

8 garlic cloves, minced

1 medium carrot, sliced

2 large sweet potatoes, scrubbed, skins left on,
and cut into ½-inch cubes

4 cups organic chicken broth

2 cups water

¼ cup freshly squeezed orange juice

½ cup nonfat sour cream

2 tablespoons honey

Salt and pepper to taste

½ bunch fresh chives, cut into ½-inch pieces

1 Heat a 4-quart saucepan over medium to medium-high heat.

2 Add the olive oil and the onion and cook for 5 minutes, stirring often.

3 Reduce the heat to medium and add the garlic. Sprinkle with 1 teaspoon salt and cook for 10 minutes, stirring often, until the onion and garlic turn light brown.

4 Add the carrot and the sweet potato, then the chicken broth and water.

5 Turn up the heat to high until it comes to a low boil again, then reduce to medium heat.

6 Leave at a slow boil, uncovered, for 45 minutes. Remove from heat and add the orange juice.

7 Ladle into a food processor and process in 4 batches until smooth. Add water in ½-cup increments up to 3 cups.

8 | As each blended soup is finished, pour back into a 4-quart saucepan over low to medium-low heat.

9 | Whisk in the sour cream and honey.

10 | Season to taste with salt and pepper and garnish with fresh chives.

Nutrient	Calories (kcal)	Carbohydrates (g)	Protein (g)	Fat (g)
Single Serving	277	38	11	9

Baked Sweet Potato and Broccoli

  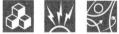

SERVES 4
90 MINUTES

8 large eggs

1 cup plain nonfat yogurt;
add pinch of salt and pepper

1 teaspoon red pepper

1 tablespoon white vinegar

3 teaspoons salt

1 teaspoon ground pepper

2 medium sweet potatoes,
peeled and diced into ½-inch pieces

1 medium head fresh broccoli

1 medium onion, coarsely chopped

1 medium yellow bell pepper, cored,
seeded, and cut into ½-inch strips

1 cup grated Monterey Jack cheese

2 tablespoons grated Parmesan cheese

1 In a large mixing bowl, beat eggs, yogurt, red pepper, vinegar, salt, and pepper until blended.

2 Place sweet potatoes in a 3-quart saucepan, cover with water, and boil for 20 minutes. Strain and set aside to cool.

3 Cut the broccoli into small florets, discarding the stalks. Place the broccoli in a 3-quart saucepan, cover with water, and boil for 20 minutes. Strain and set aside to cool.

4 Preheat the oven to 350°F.

5 Place all the ingredients except the eggs and the cheese in a 3-inch-deep rectangular glass baking dish.

6 | Pour the egg mixture over.

7 | Bake uncovered for 30 minutes.

8 | Sprinkle the cheeses on top and bake for 20 more minutes.

Nutrient	Calories (kcal)	Carbohydrates (g)	Protein (g)	Fat (g)
Single Serving	443	30	29	23

Simple Hummus Dip

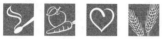

MAKES ABOUT 2 CUPS (½ CUP PER SERVING)
10 MINUTES

1 can (15 ounces) chickpeas (garbanzo beans)
1 garlic clove, minced
3 tablespoons olive oil
1 teaspoon cumin
2 tablespoons freshly squeezed lemon juice
Salt and pepper to taste

1   Drain the chickpeas and reserve the liquid.

2   Put the beans in a food processor and add the garlic, olive oil, cumin, and lemon juice.

3   Process until completely puréed, adding back the reserved liquid to achieve the desired consistency (like loose peanut butter).

4   Season to taste with salt and pepper.

NOTE: Garlic gets stronger over time. If serving immediately, use 2 cloves of garlic. If serving over a couple of days, use 1 clove.

Nutrient	Calories (kcal)	Carbohydrates (g)	Protein (g)	Fat (g)
Single Serving	438	66	21	10

Creamy Soybean Soup

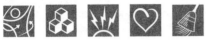

SERVES 4
2 HOURS

> 1 bag (14 ounces) frozen soybeans,
>   beans only
> 2 tablespoons unsalted butter
> 1 medium onion, diced (½ cup)
> 1 medium leek (green and white parts),
>   diced (2 cups)
> ½ small carrot, diced (¼ cup)
> 2 cups chicken broth, preferably organic
> 4 cups water
> 1 cup nonfat sour cream
> Salt and pepper to taste

1 Remove the soybeans from the freezer and let thaw.

2 Heat a 4-quart saucepan over medium heat.

3 Stir in the butter, then add the onion and leek and stir for 5 minutes.

4 Add the soybeans and carrot and stir for 1 minute.

5 Add the chicken broth and water, and turn up the heat to high until the mixture comes to a low boil, then reduce to a simmer.

6 Simmer uncovered for 45 minutes.

7 Remove from the heat and set aside for 5 minutes.

8 Separate the liquid and the soybeans and set the liquid aside.

9 In a food processor, purée ¼ of the soybeans and ¼ cup of the sour cream until smooth, adding the liquid back in as necessary until the consistency is that of a creamy soup.

10 | Continue to process until all the soup is puréed.

11 | Place back into a 4-quart saucepan and return to medium-low heat on stove top.

12 | Stir for 3 minutes and season to taste with salt and pepper.

Nutrient	Calories (kcal)	Carbohydrates (g)	Protein (g)	Fat (g)
Single Serving	599	46	43	27

Oven-Seared Chicken Breast with Black Beans and Orange Sauce

   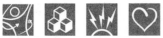

SERVES 4
2 HOURS

ORANGE SAUCE:

3 cups freshly squeezed orange juice

1 tablespoon honey

1 tablespoon jasmine or long-grain white rice

1 tablespoon cold, unsalted butter

½ teaspoon salt

1 teaspoon ground white pepper

1 | Place the orange juice, honey, and rice in a heavy-bottomed, 2-quart saucepan over medium-high heat.

2 | Bring the mixture to a slow boil.

3 | Reduce the heat so that the liquid continues to simmer slowly.

4 | Cook at a slow simmer, uncovered, for 45 minutes to 1 hour, or until liquid is reduced by two-thirds.

5 | Remove the rice from the heat and process in a food processor until the mixture is smooth.

6 | Strain and place back into the saucepan over low heat.

7 | Just before serving, turn the heat to medium and add the butter, stirring continuously until the butter has been incorporated into the sauce.

8 | Salt and pepper to taste.

4 boneless, skinless chicken breasts (6 ounces each)

3 tablespoons olive oil

Salt and pepper to taste

1 | Preheat the oven to 400°F.

2 | Put a heavy-based, 12-inch skillet in the oven.

3 | Rub the chicken breasts with the olive oil and sprinkle with salt and pepper.

4 | Using tongs, place the chicken in the hot pan.

5 | Close the oven door and cook for 20 minutes on one side, then flip and cook 20 minutes on the other side.

6 | Remove from the oven and pierce with a fork. If the juices are still a little pink, place back in the oven for 10 more minutes until juices run clear.

7 | Set aside.

BLACK BEANS:

1 can (15 ounces) whole,
    organic black beans

3 medium garlic cloves, thinly sliced

¾ cup chicken broth

1 sprig fresh thyme,
    or 1 teaspoon high-quality dried thyme

1 tablespoon olive oil

Salt and pepper to taste

1 | Drain the beans.

2 | Put all the ingredients in a 2-quart saucepan over medium heat.

3 | Simmer for 15–20 minutes, until almost all the liquid is gone.

3 green onions, thinly sliced

TO SERVE: Place a scoop of black beans in the center of the plate. Place a chicken breast on top. Pour 2 to 3 tablespoons of orange glaze over each chicken breast. Sprinkle the green onion over the top.

Nutrient	Calories (kcal)	Carbohydrates (g)	Protein (g)	Fat (g)
Single Serving	740	96	44	20

Roasted Turkey Breast with Spiced Lentils and Yogurt Curry

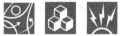

SERVES 4
1 HOUR

TURKEY:

1½ pounds boneless, skinless turkey breast,
    in one piece if possible, or use 2 breast tenderloins
4 tablespoons canola oil
Salt and pepper to taste

1   Preheat the oven to 400°F.

2   Rub the turkey with the canola oil and sprinkle with salt and pepper.

3   Place on a baking sheet or in a heavy pan (such as a cast-iron skillet).

4   Roast for 35–40 minutes.

5   Remove from the oven, pierce with a fork, and press. Make sure that the juices that flow out are clear. If still a little pink, then return to the oven for 10 more minutes. Set aside.

SPICED LENTILS:

1 cup green lentils
2 tablespoons olive oil
3 shallots, finely minced
2 garlic cloves, finely minced
1 teaspoon ground black pepper
1½ teaspoons ground cumin
½ teaspoon yellow curry powder
¼ teaspoon chili powder
2½ cups water
Salt to taste

1 | Soak the lentils in warm water for 4 hours.

2 | Drain the lentils and set aside.

3 | Heat a 4-quart saucepan over medium to medium-high heat.

4 | Add the olive oil and the shallots and stir for 3 minutes.

5 | Add the garlic and stir for 1 minute.

6 | Add the lentils and the remaining ingredients except the salt and pepper.

7 | Cook for 15–20 minutes. Season to taste with salt and pepper.

8 | Test the lentils by scooping one out with a spoon and tasting. If still firm, cook for 5 more minutes and test again, repeating until done.

YOGURT CURRY:
1 cup organic nonfat yogurt
1 tablespoon honey
3 tablespoons yellow curry powder
¼ teaspoon chili powder
½ teaspoon white pepper
1 teaspoon white wine vinegar
Salt to taste

1 | Place all the ingredients except salt in a large mixing bowl.

2 | Stir until blended and smooth.

3 | Season to taste with salt.

TO SERVE: Spoon the lentils onto the center of the plate. Slice the turkey on a cutting board. Place slices of turkey on the lentils and cover the turkey with a few tablespoons of the yogurt.

Nutrient	Calories (kcal)	Carbohydrates (g)	Protein (g)	Fat (g)
Single Serving	464	51	29	16

Broiled Salmon on Buckwheat Noodles with Ginger and Soy

SERVES 4
45 MINUTES

SALMON:

4 boneless, skinless salmon fillets (6 ounces each)

(Vegan: Substitute four 4-ounce bricks fresh tofu,
patted dry, seared in a hot nonstick pan with olive oil.
Warm in a 400°F oven for 10 minutes before serving.)

1 tablespoon olive oil

Salt and pepper

1 | Preheat the oven 450°F.

2 | Arrange the salmon on a baking sheet.

3 | Sprinkle with the olive oil, salt, and pepper.

4 | Bake for 15 minutes.

5 | Turn the broiler on high setting.

6 | Place under the broiler for 4 minutes.

NOTE: It's good to have the salmon golden brown on the top and important to cook salmon through, as it will be more tender.

NOODLES:

8 ounces buckwheat noodles

1 teaspoon salt

1 bunch green onions, root ends and ½ of the green tips removed,
sliced into thin ¼-inch rounds

¼ cup low-sodium soy sauce

¼ cup mirin (Japanese cooking wine)

3 tablespoons canola oil

2 tablespoons chopped fresh ginger, or 2 teaspoons ground ginger

1 tablespoon freshly squeezed lemon juice

1 garlic clove, minced

Salt and pepper to taste

1   Place a 3-quart saucepan ⅔ filled with water over high heat. Add 1 teaspoon salt and bring to a boil.

2   Add the noodles, return the water to a boil, then reduce to a low boil and cook for 8 minutes, until the noodles still have firmness but aren't dry and don't taste like raw flour.

3   While the noodles are cooking, place the rest of the ingredients in a mixing bowl and stir.

4   When the noodles are done, drain and toss immediately into the mixing bowl of sauce.

TO SERVE: Place the noodles and sauce in a shallow bowl. Arrange the salmon on top.

Nutrient	Calories (kcal)	Carbohydrates (g)	Protein (g)	Fat (g)
Single Serving	648	47	43	32

Red Chili and Honey Rubbed Pork Sirloin with Sweet Potato Spears

  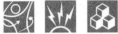

SERVES 4
45 MINUTES

PORK:

4 pork loin steaks (6 ounces each), fat trimmed off
   (Vegan: Substitute four 4-ounce bricks fresh tofu, patted dry,
   seared in a hot nonstick skillet with olive oil.)
Honey Rub (recipe follows)

1 | Preheat the oven to 400°F.

2 | Place the pork loins on a baking sheet and bake for 25–35 minutes, until desired doneness.

3 | Remove the pork loins and rub, brush, or bathe with honey rub (see below).

4 | Turn the broiler to high setting and place the pork under for 3–5 minutes.

RED CHILI AND HONEY RUB:

Also delicious when rubbed on chicken, tofu, or salmon. Can be made and put in the refrigerator, sealed, for 7 days.

½ cup honey
3 tablespoons freshly squeezed lemon juice
2 tablespoons red chili powder
1 teaspoon kosher salt
½ teaspoon freshly ground black pepper

1 | Place all the rub ingredients in a small mixing bowl and stir until well blended.

2 | Set aside to use on pork.

SWEET POTATO SPEARS:

Can be served as an accompaniment with lots of dishes or on their own.

2 medium sweet potatoes
3 tablespoons olive oil
1 sprig fresh thyme, or 1 teaspoon dried thyme
Dash salt and pepper

1 | Rinse, scrub, and dry the sweet potatoes. Cut into eighths vertically, then place in a large mixing bowl.

2 | Add the olive oil, thyme, salt, and pepper, and toss to coat the sweet potatoes.

3 | Rub a baking sheet with excess oil.

4 | Place the sweet potatoes on a baking sheet and roast in the same 400°F oven for 45 minutes, turning occasionally until soft in the middle and light brown on the outside.

OPTIONAL SALAD:

8 ounces organic baby greens
Good Basic Salad Dressing (page 65)

Toss the greens in salad dressing as needed and set aside.

TO SERVE: Arrange the sweet potato spears on individual serving plates. Place the optional salad on the spears. Place the pork on top and serve.

Nutrient	Calories (kcal)	Carbohydrates (g)	Protein (g)	Fat (g)
Single Serving	478	35	35	22

Cumin-Basted Pork Loin with Rosemary Polenta and Creamy Leeks

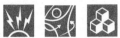

SERVES 4
1¼ HOURS

PORK:

1 pound lean pork loin, trimmed of all fat

Cumin Basting Sauce (recipe follows)

1 Preheat the oven to 375°F.

2 Rub the pork with the cumin basting sauce (see below) and place on a heavy baking sheet.

3 Roast for 30–35 minutes.

4 Poke with the tip of a knife; if juice runs clear, then it's cooked to medium-well; if it's slightly pink, it's medium; and if there is no liquid, it's beyond well. Cook to desired doneness.

5 Remove from the heat and let rest for 5–10 minutes before slicing.

CUMIN BASTING SAUCE:

2 tablespoons ground cumin

2 tablespoons brown sugar

2 garlic cloves, minced

1 teaspoon ground ginger

1 teaspoon salt

1 teaspoon ground black pepper

1 teaspoon water

1 tablespoon olive oil

1 | Heat a nonstick skillet over medium-low heat.

2 | Add the cumin to the dry pan and stir continuously until the slightest amount of smoke and aroma comes off the pan.

3 | Remove from the heat and set aside to cool.

4 | Stir all the sauce ingredients, including the cumin, together in a medium-size mixing bowl.

POLENTA:

3 cups water
¾ cup yellow cornmeal
3 sprigs fresh rosemary, finely chopped,
    or 3 teaspoons dried rosemary
¼ cup nonfat or low-fat sour cream
2 tablespoons unsalted butter
Salt and pepper to taste

1 | Place a 3-quart saucepan over high heat. Add the water, bring to a boil, and turn down heat to medium. Sprinkle in the cornmeal ⅓ at a time, stirring constantly with a whisk at first, then as it thickens with a wooden spoon. When it starts to thicken (about 5 minutes), add the rosemary, reduce heat, and let bubble for 5 minutes.

2 | Remove from the heat and stir in the sour cream and the butter.

3 | Season to taste with salt and pepper.

NOTE: The longer the polenta sits, the stiffer it will get and you may need to add up to 1 cup more water and reheat. If so, you must reseason after each addition of water.

CREAMY LEEKS:

3 tablespoons cold, unsalted butter, cut into ½-inch cubes
3 large leeks, root end and 1 inch of green tips removed, sliced into ¼-inch rounds
Salt and pepper to taste

1. Place a 3-quart saucepan over low to medium heat, add the butter, then add the leeks. Cook for 15 minutes, stirring occasionally, until the leeks still have their bright color but are spaghetti soft. Do not let brown or burn.

2. Add salt and pepper to taste.

3. Remove from pan; set aside to keep warm.

TO SERVE: Spoon polenta onto serving plate. Top with leeks. Slice the pork into ¼-inch slices and lay on top. If you have fresh rosemary sprigs left over, use them for a garnish.

Nutrient	Calories (kcal)	Carbohydrates (g)	Protein (g)	Fat (g)
Single Serving	534	39	27	30

Russet Potato and Green Onion Soup

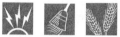

SERVES 4

45 MINUTES

4 large russet potatoes, scrubbed, skins left on,
 and cut into 6 pieces

1 small yellow onion, coarsely chopped

1 small garlic clove, peeled

1 teaspoon salt

1 cup 1 percent or nonfat milk

½ stick unsalted butter

1 bunch green onions, thinly sliced

3 tablespoons grated Parmesan cheese

1 Place a 5-quart saucepan with the potatoes, onions, garlic, and salt over high heat, bring to a boil, and reduce to a low boil for 20–25 minutes, or until the potatoes are soft but not mushy.

2 Add the milk and bring to a boil.

3 Remove from the heat and add butter.

4 Let the soup cool for a few minutes.

5 Purée the cooled soup in a food processor in two batches until smooth.

6 Stir in the green onion.

7 Sprinkle with the grated Parmesan before serving.

Nutrient	Calories (kcal)	Carbohydrates (g)	Protein (g)	Fat (g)	Total Dietary Fiber (g)
Single Serving	269	26	12	13	10

Pasta Salad with Chicken and Black Olive Pesto

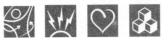

SERVES 4
35 MINUTES

CHICKEN:

2 boneless, skinless chicken breasts (6 ounces each)
    (Vegan: Substitute two 4-ounce bricks of fresh tofu.
    After searing in a pan, roast for 10 minutes only.)
1 tablespoon olive oil
Salt and pepper to taste

1 | Preheat the oven 450°F.

2 | Arrange the chicken breasts on a baking sheet and sprinkle with the olive oil, salt, and pepper.

3 | Bake for 15–18 minutes, until chicken is no longer pink in the center.

4 | Preheat the broiler on high setting and broil the chicken for 3–5 minutes, until golden brown.

5 | Remove the chicken from the broiler and let cool, then pull the chicken into ½-inch strips.

PASTA:

1 pound rotini or penne pasta
1 teaspoon salt
1 tablespoon olive oil

1 | Place a 3-quart saucepan filled ⅔ with water over high heat and add 1 teaspoon salt.

2 | When boiling, add the pasta, stir, and reduce the heat to a low boil.

3 | Boil for 6 minutes. Pull a piece of pasta out, set on a plate, and let cool for a minute. If it has texture but doesn't taste raw, it's done.

4 | Turn off the burner and remove the pasta.

5 | Drain and run cool water over the pasta for 5 minutes.

6 | Toss the pasta with the olive oil in a large mixing bowl and set aside.

PESTO:

1 bunch basil

½ cup pitted kalamata olives

¼ cup pine nuts

3 tablespoons grated Parmesan cheese

3 tablespoons olive oil

2 tablespoons water

1 teaspoon red chili powder

Place all the pesto ingredients in a blender and process on high speed until a fine but slightly chunky sauce forms.

TO SERVE: When the pasta comes out of the water cooked and drained and cooled, toss with the chicken and pesto in a large mixing bowl. Serve while cool, not cold. Season with salt, if desired.

Nutrient	Calories (kcal)	Carbohydrates (g)	Protein (g)	Fat (g)
Single Serving	646	73	32	25

Chilled Watermelon Soup

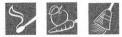

SERVES 4
25 MINUTES

½ small seedless watermelon,
 peeled and cut into 2-inch pieces
½ cup honey
½ cup cranberry juice
4 fresh mint sprigs (optional)

1   Place all the ingredients except mint in a food processor and process on high until the mixture is smooth.

2   Place in the refrigerator to chill.

3   Serve in bowls and add a sprig of mint to each serving.

Nutrient	Calories (kcal)	Carbohydrates (g)	Protein (g)	Fat (g)
Single Serving	342	77	4	2

Mellow Jean's Yellow Pepper Soup

4 SERVINGS
50 MINUTES

3 large yellow peppers, cored and seeded

1 small yellow onion, cored

1 medium carrot, cut into ¼-inch rounds

2 tablespoons olive oil

1 cup vegetable broth (or water)

4 cups water

½ teaspoon yellow curry, optional

2 tablespoons honey

¾ cup nonfat sour cream

Salt and pepper to taste

1   Cut each pepper into six pieces. Cut each onion in half, then cut each half into eight pieces. Place all ingredients except the sour cream, honey, and salt and pepper in a 5-quart saucepan over high heat.

2   Bring to a boil, and reduce heat to a low boil for 35 minutes.

3   Remove from heat and purée in a food processor in batches until smooth.

4   Strain with a medium-fine mesh strainer back into the saucepan. This step is optional; the result will be chunkier and slightly more tart if not strained.

5   Discard pulp.

6   Place sour cream in a bowl with the honey, and whisk in ½ cup of the soup mixture to blend.

7   Place soup over medium-high heat and stir in sour cream and honey mixture.

8   Season with salt and pepper to taste.

Nutrient	Calories (kcal)	Carbohydrates (g)	Protein (g)	Fat (g)
Single Serving	245	35	6	9

Snack Bar with Nuts and Raisins

MAKES ENOUGH FOR 12 BARS
1 HOUR, PLUS TIME TO SET UP

1 cup cashews

1 cup unsalted raw peanuts

1 cup walnuts

1 cup almonds

½ cup pine nuts

1 cup raisins

1 cup pitted dates

½ cup currants

½ cup prunes

½ cup unsulfured dried apricots

1 cup rolled oats

1 cup oat bran

¼ cup wheat germ

½ cup organic chocolate morsels

¼ cup cocoa powder

2 tablespoons unrefined brown sugar/evaporated cane juice

1½ cups warm water mixed with 3 tablespoons honey

1   Grind all the ingredients except the water and honey mixture in a food processor.

2   Place the mixture in a large mixing bowl.

3   Stir in the water and honey mixture with a wooden spoon. Add ¼ cup more water if needed.

4   Line a loaf pan with plastic wrap, with edges of wrap overhanging pan.

5   Form the mixture in loaf pan and let set for 45 minutes.

6 | Use the plastic wrap to lift loaf from pan.

7 | Cut into slices to serve.

8 | Keep tightly wrapped and refrigerated.

Nutrient	Calories (kcal)	Carbohydrates (g)	Protein (g)	Fat (g)
Single Serving	703	82	19	33

One-Pan Chicken and Legume Stir-Fry

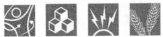

SERVES 4
1 HOUR

RICE:

1 cup uncooked brown rice
½ small onion, minced
2 tablespoons canola oil
1½ cups water
Salt and pepper to taste

1 | Place a 2-quart saucepan over medium-high heat.

2 | Add the canola oil.

3 | Add the onion and stir continuously for 3 minutes.

4 | Add the rice and stir for 30 seconds.

5 | Add the water.

6 | Bring to a boil.

7 | Reduce to a simmer, cover, and cook until all the water is absorbed, stirring occasionally.

8 | Remove the rice from the heat, fluff up with a spoon, and season with salt and pepper to taste.

STIR-FRY:

1 pound boneless, skinless chicken breast, sliced into thin strips
4 tablespoons arrowroot
4 tablespoons canola oil
½ small onion, sliced into thin strips
1 leek, thinly sliced
1 medium red bell pepper, cored, seeded, and thinly sliced

1 medium yellow bell pepper, cored, seeded, and thinly sliced

½ cup snow peas, sliced into thin strips

1 garlic clove, minced

3 tablespoons low-sodium soy sauce

1 tablespoon freshly squeezed lemon juice

2 teaspoons minced fresh ginger

Salt and pepper to taste

1. On a flat baking sheet, roll the chicken in arrowroot until covered.

2. Heat a large nonstick pan or wok over medium-high heat.

3. Add 3 tablespoons of the canola oil.

4. Add the chicken and cook, stirring, for 5–7 minutes.

5. Set aside until the vegetable mixture is finished.

6. Heat a separate large nonstick pan or wok over medium-high heat.

7. Add the remaining 1 tablespoon of canola oil.

8. Add the onion and cook, stirring for 3 minutes.

9. Add the leek and bell peppers and cook, stirring, for 3 minutes.

10. Add the snow peas and the garlic and cook, stirring, for 7 minutes.

11. Stir in the rest of the ingredients, then stir in the cooked chicken.

12. Season to taste.

TO SERVE: Make a well of rice in the center of the plate. Fill it with the stir-fry mixture.

Nutrient	Calories (kcal)	Carbohydrates (g)	Protein (g)	Fat (g)
Single Serving	533	53	33	21

Bonito Burritos

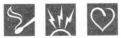

SERVES 4
15 MINUTES

4 large organic sprouted-wheat tortillas
½ cup grated Monterey Jack cheese
1 ripe organic tomato (beefsteak or similar size),
    cut into small cubes
Pinch kosher salt
2 cups organic baby spinach, trimmed and sliced thinly
    or ripped up into small pieces
1 ripe avocado, peeled and cubed
Hot sauce to taste (optional)

1   Preheat the broiler on high setting.

2   Lay out all tortillas on a baking sheet.

3   Spread the cheese on one half and the diced tomato on the other half of the open tortilla.

4   Sprinkle a pinch of salt on the tomato.

5   Place under the broiler for 5 minutes, or until the cheese is fully melted.

6   When fully melted, place the spinach and avocado on the tortilla.

7   Add the optional hot sauce.

8   Roll up and place under the broiler for 3 more minutes.

Nutrient	Calories (kcal)	Carbohydrates (g)	Protein (g)	Fat (g)
Single Serving	289	34	9	13

Roasted Citrus-Stuffed Chicken with Couscous

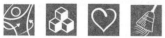

SERVES 4
1½ HOURS

CHICKEN:

1 roasting chicken (5 pounds), cleaned

1 teaspoon salt

2 lemons, rubbed on a fine grater to remove the outer layer of the peel,
   which should yield about 1 teaspoon
   (reserve for the couscous), then halved

1 orange, quartered

1 lime, halved

4 garlic cloves, halved

Salt and pepper

1 Preheat the oven to 400°F.

2 Sprinkle the 1 teaspoon salt inside the chicken and stuff with the citrus and garlic.

3 Sprinkle the outside with salt and pepper.

4 Place in a roasting pan and roast for 1¼ hours, or until liquid runs clear from the cavity.

5 Squeeze the juice of the extra citrus over the top.

COUSCOUS:

2 tablespoons olive oil

½ small onion, cut into ¼-inch pieces

1½ cups couscous

2 cups water

Zest of 2 lemons (see above)

1 tablespoon freshly squeezed lemon juice

1 teaspoon dried mint

1 teaspoon white pepper

1 cup fresh baby spinach, rinsed and dried

1   While the chicken is cooking, place a 3-quart saucepan over medium heat and add oil.

2   Add the onion and stir constantly for 2 minutes.

3   Add the couscous and stir constantly for 1 minute.

4   Turn the heat to high.

5   Add the water and boil for 2 minutes. Turn off the heat and set aside for 8 minutes.

6   Fluff with a fork and add the rest of the ingredients just before serving.

TO SERVE: Make a mound of the couscous in a bowl, and serve the chicken on a platter.

Nutrient	Calories (kcal)	Carbohydrates (g)	Protein (g)	Fat (g)
Single Serving	976	65	116	28

Sweet Potato Mash

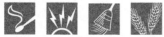

MAKES 4 GENEROUS SERVINGS
45 MINUTES

3 medium sweet potatoes, scrubbed, skins left on,
and cut into 2-inch pieces
1 small onion, halved, each half cut into 3 pieces
2 teaspoons salt
1 tablespoon unsalted butter
1 tablespoon olive oil
(Vegan: Use 2 tablespoons olive oil instead of
1 tablespoon each butter and olive oil.)
Salt and pepper to taste

1 Place a 4-quart saucepan over high heat and add potatoes and onions, enough water to cover them by 2 inches, and 2 teaspoons of the salt.

2 Bring to a boil, then turn to a low boil for 25 minutes, until the sweet potatoes are soft when tested with a fork.

3 Remove from the heat and drain, leaving ½ cup of cooking water.

4 While still warm fork-mash the sweet potatoes with the butter, olive oil, salt, and pepper. The mash can be rustic and chunky. Stir in the reserved cooking water to reach the desired consistency.

NOTE: Potatoes eat up the salt flavor over time, so always taste before serving and adjust seasoning as needed.

TO SERVE: Use as a side dish, as a base for a tuna steak (page 38), or chill overnight, form into cakes, and sear in oil in a skillet to serve with your morning eggs.

Nutrient	Calories (kcal)	Carbohydrates (g)	Protein (g)	Fat (g)
Single Serving	171	25	2	7

KEY FOODS AND RECIPES FOR THE TRANSITION PERIOD

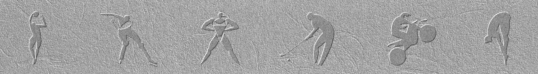

THE TRANSITION PERIOD SHOULD BE A PART OF EVERY ACTIVE PERSON'S year. For competitive athletes, it provides a time for unstructured exercise, mental relaxation, and physical recuperation. For more fitness- and wellness-oriented people, it's the time of the year when you're least active, either because of other commitments, weather, daylight hours, or other interests. In either case, the Transition Period features a healthy and much-needed reduction in training volume and intensity, which allows your body and mind to relax, reflect, and refocus on new goals.

At the same time, you shouldn't mistake the Transition Period with a prolonged vacation from exercise. If you were to stop exercising completely for a month, it would take you another two months just to regain the fitness you lost. It is difficult to make significant progress from one year to the next when you spend three months losing and regaining fitness.

The goal of training in the Transition Period is to maintain your aerobic conditioning. You've spent so much time building your aerobic engine, it would be a shame to let that fitness disappear. Fortunately, it doesn't take a huge amount of training to prevent the aerobic system from detraining. Your weekly training hours can be about 25 percent less than what they were during the Foundation Period, and you will still get through the Transition Period with the majority of your aerobic capacity intact. Instead of sitting on the couch for weeks, reduce your training volume and intensity and take the regimen out of training. If you normally train five days each week, add another rest day. Spend time participating in different sports than you normally would.

Feeding the Transition Period

Since the volume and intensity of the Transition Period are lower than during any other portion of the year, your caloric intake needs to decrease. You're not burning as much energy on a daily basis, and if you continue eating as if you are, you will quickly gain unnecessary weight. Gaining a few pounds is normal, and even recommended, but you should aim to keep this weight gain to about 5–7 pounds (2–3 kilograms).

Making the transition from the highest caloric intake of the year (Specialization Period) to the lowest (Transition Period) can be challenging. The changes in your eating habits and portion sizes should be gradual over the period of one to two weeks, rather than a sudden reduction over a few days. One way to ease this transition is to start incorporating foods that are high in fiber and relatively low in calories. Fiber makes a food filling, meaning you feel satiated sooner, even though you've consumed fewer calories.

The Transition Period is the one part of the year when slightly restricting carbohydrate intake may be beneficial to an active individual. It's not so much a matter of avoiding carbohydrate to prevent it from being converted to and stored as fat. Rather, it's a matter of consuming the appropriate amount of carbohydrate in relation to the amount of activity you're involved in. During the Preparation and Specialization periods, a lot of emphasis was put on carbohydrate because your activity level demanded it. In the Transition and Foundation periods, your lower activity level places a higher emphasis on balance, and it is not as necessary to seek additional sources of concentrated carbohydrate energy.

If there is any fuel that receives more attention during the Transition Period, it's protein. Not only do high-protein foods tend to be satiating, which helps in controlling energy intake, but also your body is in a period of recuperation. Protein is essential for building and repairing muscle and connective tissues (tendons and ligaments), and there is a lot of repair work happening during this period. Your immune system also takes advantage of this period of reduced stress to adapt and fortify itself in preparation for harder days ahead. If you look back at the tables on pages 10–11, you'll see that the recommended protein intake in the Transition Period is equal to that of the Preparation Period, even though the total daily caloric intake is significantly lower.

Key Transition Period Foods

In the process of identifying key foods for the Transition Period, I looked for items that were both nutrient-dense and filling. Active people are in the habit of eating until they are full, which serves them well during periods of high-energy intake. However, during times when energy demands are lower, these same habits make it difficult to reduce caloric intake. Consuming foods that are higher in fiber and protein, such as legumes, citrus fruits, and low-fat dairy foods, is helpful because people feel full, and consequently stop eating, after consuming fewer total calories. As a result, we can keep the typical and healthy Transition Period weight gain to just a few pounds, rather than the 15-pound spare tire some people strap on every year.

Legumes

Time to break out the beans. Black beans, pintos, garbanzo, lentils, black-eyed peas, and soybeans should be part of your nutrition program year round, and especially during the Transition Period. Besides being a good source of carbohydrate energy, they are also high in protein and fiber. What's more, legumes are lower in total fat and saturated fat than most other protein sources, including red meat and poultry. This means they contain fewer total calories than an equal-weight portion of meat or poultry.

Citrus Fruits

Citrus fruits are another group of foods that should be part of your nutrition program throughout the year. The reason they are a key food for the Transition Period is their high fiber content and the amount of vitamin C and beta-carotene they contain. Of course, in order to get the fiber from a citrus fruit, you have to eat the flesh of the fruit, as well as drinking the juice. This is often difficult to incorporate into recipes, but if you use juice that still has pulp in it for recipes that call for fruit juice, you still get a portion of the fiber from the original fruit.

Incidentally, citrus fruits are also the perfect travel food. When I used to travel all over the world as an athlete, I had to be careful to avoid food-borne illnesses. One of the ways my teammates and I stayed healthy was to pack our bags with, or purchase, citrus fruits like oranges, grapefruit, and kiwis. Basically, the rule of thumb was that if you had to peel it yourself, it was safe to eat, no matter where you were. Bananas, even though they're not citrus, fit into this category as well.

Low-Fat Dairy Products

Dairy products are exceptional sources of protein, and they tend to be quite filling. Along with the high-quality protein found in milk, yogurt, cottage cheese, and other cheeses, these foods are also excellent sources of calcium, vitamins A and D, choline, phosphorus, and vitamin B_{12}. The table below provides the nutritional features of several dairy choices.

Milk, Yogurt, Cottage Cheese Products (8-oz serving)	Calories	Fat (g)	Calcium (mg)	Vitamin A (IU)
Nonfat cottage cheese	160	0	160	400
Skim milk	80	0.4	300	16
Yogurt, skim	127	0.4	200	16
Lowfat buttermilk	98	2	285	81
1% fat cottage cheese	162	2	140	85
1% chocolate milk	143	2	285	453
1% milk	102	2	300	500
Lowfat yogurt, fruit	232	2	300	104
Soy milk	130	4	40	78
Nonfat frozen yogurt	200	5	600	400
Cottage cheese	240	10	160	400
Goat's milk	168	10	325	451
Sheep's milk	245	16	472	333
Frozen yogurt	400	9	500	400
Chocolate ice cream (Häagen-Dazs)	540	18	300	1,000

Calcium is a mineral of key importance for active people, although many do not consume nearly enough. Recommended calcium intakes are listed in the table below. Calcium is the primary mineral responsible for strong bones, but it also plays an important role in muscle contraction. During periods of strenuous exercise, your body may actually rob calcium from your bones so it can use it in muscles. This only exacerbates the challenge of maintaining bone density as you get older.

Daily Reference Intakes (DRI) for calcium according to age and gender*

1,300 mg for ages 9–18
1,000 mg for adults aged 19–50
1,200 mg for older adults
1,500 mg for postmenopausal women not taking hormone replacement therapy

*The Upper Intake Level (UL) for calcium is 2,500 mg per day. Intakes above 1,500 mg per day have not been associated with any greater benefits than more moderate intakes in the 1,200–1,500 mg per day range.

Athletes in non-weight-bearing sports like cycling and swimming face even greater challenges regarding bone density. Bones, like other tissues in the body, respond to stress. When you spend time carrying your body weight or applying stress to your skeleton through weight lifting, you encourage the deposition of calcium into bones to make them stronger. Cyclists and swimmers apply very little stress to their bones, so consequently they tend to have lower bone density. Some preliminary research has revealed that some elite cyclists in their twenties have the bone density of sixty-year-old men.

While adequate calcium intake is an important component of bone health, weight-bearing activity is as well. For a long time I've encouraged athletes in non-weight-bearing sports to run, lift weights, or play basketball or racquet sports in the Transition Period and other portions of the year in order to provide more opportunity for calcium deposition in bone. Recently, research is suggesting that short bouts of plyometric exercise (leaping, bounding, box jumps, etc.) are very effective for maintaining, and possibly increasing, bone density as well.

Red Lentil and Carrot Soup

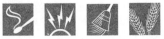

SERVES 4
ABOUT 1 HOUR

SOUP:

3 cups water

½ cup dried red lentils

2 tablespoons extra-virgin olive oil

2 large onions, chopped in ½-inch chunks

3–4 large carrots, cut in ½-inch chunks

2 tablespoons raw honey

¼ cup freshly squeezed orange juice

5 cups fresh water

Kosher or sea salt and freshly ground pepper to taste

1 Boil the 3 cups of water in a 2- to 3-quart saucepan, add the red lentils, and set aside to soak for 30 minutes.

2 Drain and set aside.

3 Heat a 4-quart saucepan over medium-high heat.

4 Add the olive oil and heat for 1 minute.

5 Add the chopped onion and stir over medium-high heat for 5 minutes.

6 Add the chopped carrot and stir for 2 minutes.

7 Add the soaked lentils, honey, orange juice, and 5 cups water and simmer over low heat for 35 minutes, until the carrots are soft.

8 Place the mixture in a food processor and process in batches until smooth.

9 Pour back into the saucepan, reheat, and season with salt and pepper to taste.

1 tablespoon molasses

1 tablespoon water

1 tablespoon finely chopped fresh tarragon

Kosher or sea salt to taste

1 Mix the molasses, water, and tarragon together until blended, and season with salt.

2 Ladle the soup into a bowl and use a spoon to drizzle the topping on top.

Nutrient	Calories (kcal)	Carbohydrates (g)	Protein (g)	Fat (g)
Single Serving	292	47	8	8

Black Bean and Toasted Cumin Dip

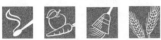

MAKES ABOUT 3 CUPS (½ CUP PER SERVING)
ABOUT 10 MINUTES

2 tablespoons ground cumin

2 cans (8 ounces each) organic black beans

¼ onion, finely chopped

3 large garlic cloves

½ teaspoon black pepper

1 teaspoon red chili powder

½ cup low-fat or nonfat sour cream

½ bunch cilantro, roughly chopped

Kosher or sea salt and pepper to taste

2 green onions, sliced, for garnish

1   Heat a nonstick skillet over medium-low heat. Add the cumin to a dry skillet, stirring continuously until the slightest amount of smoke and aroma come off the pan.

2   Place all the ingredients, including the cumin, except the green onion in a large food processor and process until smooth.

3   Serve in a bowl sprinkled with the sliced green onion. The dip can be kept, refrigerated, for up to 3 days.

Nutrient	Calories (kcal)	Carbohydrates (g)	Protein (g)	Fat (g)	Total Dietary Fiber (g)
Single Serving	312	51	18	4	12

Green Bean and Chickpea Salad

SERVES 4
ABOUT 25 MINUTES

2 teaspoons salt (preferably kosher or sea salt)

2 pounds fresh green beans, trimmed and cut into 3-inch pieces,
   or 2 bags (1 pound each) frozen organic green beans,
   thawed and drained of excess water

1 can (10 ounces) chickpeas (garbanzo beans), drained

Lemon Feta Vinaigrette (page 85)

1   Fill a large mixing bowl about halfway with ice and water.

2   Place a 3-quart saucepan ⅔ filled with water and 2 teaspoons of salt over high
   heat. When water comes to a boil, add the green beans.

3   Boil uncovered for 3–5 minutes, or until the beans still have texture but don't
   taste raw.

4   Remove the beans from the heat, drain, and immediately place into the ice water
   to stop the cooking.

5   Let stand in ice water for 10 minutes, then drain.

6   Combine the green beans with the chickpeas in a large mixing bowl.

7   Pour in the Lemon Feta Vinaigrette and toss.

Nutrient*	Calories (kcal)	Carbohydrates (g)	Protein (g)	Fat (g)
Single Serving	169	32	8	1

*Vinaigrette not included in these numbers.

Spicy Cottage Cheese

SERVES 4
5 MINUTES

16 ounces nonfat cottage cheese

3 tablespoons low-sodium soy sauce

1 tablespoon Tabasco sauce

2 garlic cloves, finely chopped

1 teaspoon minced fresh ginger or ¼ teaspoon ground ginger

¼ bunch fresh chives, thinly sliced

1 | Place all the ingredients except chives in a large mixing bowl, stir, and top with chives.

Nutrient	Calories (kcal)	Carbohydrates (g)	Protein (g)	Fat (g)
Single Serving	105	4	20	1

Cranberry and Kiwi Yogurt

SERVES 4
15 MINUTES

> 4 medium kiwifruit, peeled
>
> 16 ounces organic nonfat yogurt
>
> ½ cup cranberry juice
>
> 4 tablespoons honey
>
> 2 tablespoons maple syrup
>
> 2 tablespoons oat bran
>
> 2 tablespoons rolled oats

1 Peel and slice the kiwifruit, reserving 4 slices for garnish, then chop the rest into medium dice.

2 Place all the ingredients except the garnish in a food processor and process until smooth.

3 Serve in bowls garnished with the slices of kiwifruit.

Nutrient	Calories (kcal)	Carbohydrates (g)	Protein (g)	Fat (g)
Single Serving	241	54	4	1

Four-Egg Frittata with Black Olives, Roasted Red Pepper, Spinach, and Parmesan

SERVES 2
35 MINUTES

1 small red bell pepper, cored, seeded,
    and cut into 4 pieces

1 tablespoon olive oil

3 large egg whites and 1 large egg,
    beaten in a small mixing bowl
    with a pinch of salt and pepper

¼ cup fresh spinach, stemmed and torn into small pieces

2 tablespoons fresh basil, torn into medium-size pieces

4 black olives, pitted and quartered

Pinch salt and pepper

¼ cup grated Parmesan cheese

1 | Preheat the broiler on high setting.

2 | Place the red peppers skin side up on a baking sheet and under the broiler.

3 | When the skin of the peppers is dark brown and black, remove from the broiler, place in a small mixing bowl, and cover with plastic wrap. Set aside to cool.

4 | Remove the skin from the peppers and slice into ¼-inch strips.

5 | Place a small ovenproof nonstick sauté pan over medium-high heat and add the olive oil.

6 | When hot, add the egg mixture and stir for 1 minute until the eggs begin to very loosely come together; do not scramble.

7 | Turn the heat down to medium.

8 | Add the remaining ingredients except the Parmesan and stir once.

9 | Turn the heat down to medium for 30–40 seconds.

10 | Place under the broiler for 30 seconds, until the top is light tan.

11 | Sprinkle with the Parmesan and serve.

Nutrient	Calories (kcal)	Carbohydrates (g)	Protein (g)	Fat (g)
Single Serving	228	6	15	16

Frittata with Oven-Dried Tomato

SERVES 1
25 MINUTES

1 tablespoon olive oil

1 large egg and 2 large egg whites, beaten

1 ounce skim-milk mozzarella cheese

1 oven-dried Roma tomato

3 kalamata olives, pitted and quartered

Italian parsley

Salt and black pepper to taste

OVEN-DRIED ROMA (PLUM) TOMATOES:

This can be done once a month with four times the amount of tomato. They make a nice addition to pasta as well. Store, covered, in the refrigerator.

1 | Preheat the oven to 200°F.

2 | Place the thin tomato slices on a wire cooling rack and set on a baking sheet.

3 | Bake for 1 hour, until the tomato is dry and starting to darken on the edges.

4 | Remove from the oven and set aside to cool.

FRITTATA:

1 | Preheat the broiler on high setting.

2 | Place a small ovenproof sauté pan over medium-high heat.

3 | Add the oil when the pan is hot.

4 | Pour the eggs in and stir until 40 percent of the eggs are solidifying, then turn down heat to medium.

5 | Place the cheese on top and cook for 2 minutes.

6 Place under the broiler for 1 minute.

7 Sprinkle with the oven-dried tomato and olives, and place under the broiler for 20 more seconds.

8 Garnish with the parsley leaves and serve.

9 Season with salt and black pepper to taste.

Nutrient	Calories (kcal)	Carbohydrates (g)	Protein (g)	Fat (g)
Single Serving	219	8	22	11

Scrambled Tofu with Green Onion and Mushroom

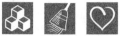

SERVES 4
30 MINUTES

1 tablespoon canola oil

1 cup diced portobello or button mushrooms

1 large red bell pepper, cored, seeded, and cut into ½-inch pieces

1 garlic clove, minced

4 green onions, thinly sliced

1 brick (4 ounces) fresh tofu block, drained, patted dry, and cubed

2 tablespoons low-sodium soy sauce

½ teaspoon toasted sesame oil (optional)

Salt to taste

1 Place a large sauté pan over medium-high heat. When hot, add the canola oil.

2 Add the mushrooms, peppers, and garlic, and raise the heat to high for 1 minute, stirring often.

3 Lower the heat to medium-high and stir occasionally for 5 minutes.

4 Add the green onion and stir 1 minute.

5 Lower to just below medium heat and add the rest of the ingredients, stirring once.

6 Cook for 3 minutes.

7 Season with more soy sauce and toasted sesame oil as desired.

Nutrient	Calories (kcal)	Carbohydrates (g)	Protein (g)	Fat (g)
Single Serving	199	10	15	11

Pan-Roasted Chicken Breast with Cranberry Glaze and Roasted Sweet Potatoes

 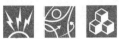

SERVES 4
1 HOUR

CHICKEN:

4 boneless, skinless chicken breasts (6 ounces each)
    (Vegan: Substitute four 4-ounce bricks fresh tofu.
    After searing in a pan, roast for 10 minutes only.
    Don't broil.)
1 tablespoon olive oil
Salt and pepper

1 | Preheat the oven to 450°F.

2 | While the chicken and sweet potato are cooking, start cranberry glaze.

3 | Arrange the chicken breasts on a baking sheet and sprinkle with olive oil, salt, and pepper.

5 | Bake for 15–18 minutes, until the chicken is no longer pink in the middle.

6 | Preheat the broiler on high setting, and broil for 3–5 minutes, until golden brown.

7 | Remove from broiler.

POTATOES:

These can be done a day in advance and reheated in the oven at 400°F for 10 minutes.

3 medium sweet potatoes, washed,
    skins left on, cut into 8 pieces
2 tablespoons olive oil
2 teaspoons salt
1 teaspoon pepper

1 | Preheat the oven to 450°F.

2 | Place a 3-quart saucepan over high heat, add potatoes, and fill with water to cover 2 inches over the top of the potatoes.

3 | Boil until the potatoes are semisoft to the fork, then remove the pan from heat and drain the potatoes.

4 | Place in a large mixing bowl and toss with the olive oil, salt, and pepper.

5 | Spread on a baking sheet and bake for 15 minutes, or until golden brown.

6 | Remove from the oven and set aside.

OPTIONAL:

1 | After the sweet potatoes have been boiled and roasted, place in a large mixing bowl.

2 | Add ¾ stick unsalted butter, 1 teaspoon salt, and 1 tablespoon brown sugar.

3 | Mash with a large fork until rough and rustic-looking.

4 | Use as a bed for the chicken.

CRANBERRY GLAZE, EZ WAY:

½ jar (6- or 8-ounce size) cranberry sauce
3 tablespoons freshly squeezed orange juice
1 tablespoon unsalted butter
Salt to taste

Place all the ingredients in a saucepan and warm and stir before serving.

NOT AS EZ WAY:

1 8-ounce bag frozen or fresh cranberries
½ orange, peeled and cut in segments
1 cup freshly squeezed orange juice
¼ cup and 2 tablespoons honey
½ stick unsalted butter
Salt to taste

1 | Place all the ingredients except the unsalted butter and salt in a 3-quart saucepan over low to medium heat and simmer for 30 minutes.

2 | When mixture starts to thicken, stir in the butter and season with salt.

3 | Pour over the chicken to serve.

Nutrient*	Calories (kcal)	Carbohydrates (g)	Protein (g)	Fat (g)
Single Serving	388	37	33	12

*Numbers reflect recipe made with EZ cranberry glaze.

Black Bean and Roasted Chicken Chili

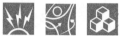

SERVES 4
1¼ HOURS

2 boneless, skinless chicken breasts (6 ounces each),
  cut into ½-inch strips

2 cans (8 ounces each) black beans

2 cups chicken broth

2 cups cool water

1 medium onion, coarsely chopped

2 garlic cloves, minced as finely as possible

2 ounces tequila

1 tablespoon cumin seed, toasted

1 tablespoon chopped fresh oregano, or 1 teaspoon dried oregano

1 tablespoon red chili powder

1 tablespoon white distilled vinegar

1 teaspoon unsweetened cocoa powder

Salt to taste

TO FINISH:

½ cup chopped cilantro

1 tablespoon freshly squeezed lime juice

1 teaspoon salt

1 Place all the ingredients except the finish in a 5-quart saucepan over medium heat for 50 minutes.

2 Stir in the finish just before serving.

Nutrient	Calories (kcal)	Carbohydrates (g)	Protein (g)	Fat (g)
Single Serving	565	79	51	5

Turkey Tacos Over Green Chili Polenta

SERVES 4
40 MINUTES

TURKEY TACO MIX:

3 tablespoons ground cumin

1 tablespoon red chili powder

2 tablespoons olive oil

1 small yellow onion, diced

1½ pounds ground turkey breast

1 teaspoon ground black pepper

Salt to taste

1 Place a nonstick pan over medium heat, add ground cumin and red chili powder, and stir for 3 minutes. Remove from heat and set aside to cool.

2 Place a large sauté pan over medium-high heat and add oil when hot.

3 Add the onion and stir for 3 minutes.

4 Add the cooled chili powder and cumin and stir for 1 minute.

5 Add the ground turkey, turn the heat to medium, and stir occasionally until cooked through.

6 Season to taste with salt and pepper.

GREEN CHILI POLENTA:

You can use this to serve with tofu or cod fillets.

4 cups water

1 cup yellow cornmeal

1 teaspoon salt

1 medium poblano or Anaheim chili pepper, cored, seeded, and cut into ¼-inch pieces

½ cup nonfat sour cream

Salt and pepper to taste

1 | Place the 4 cups of water in a 4-quart saucepan and set over high heat.

2 | Bring to a boil, then reduce to a low boil.

3 | Sprinkle the cornmeal into the boiling water 1 tablespoon at time, first stirring with a whisk, then, as it thickens, with a wooden spoon.

4 | Once all the cornmeal is incorporated, lower heat and let bubble for 3–5 minutes, stirring occasionally.

5 | Remove from the heat and stir in the remaining ingredients. If it is too thick, add a little more water until creamy.

TO SERVE: Place a scoop of polenta in a bowl. Spoon the turkey taco mix over.

VARIATION: Scoop the turkey taco mix into taco shells with a little shredded lettuce.

Nutrient	Calories (kcal)	Carbohydrates (g)	Protein (g)	Fat (g)
Single Serving	419	33	47	11

Ricotta and Spinach Lasagna

 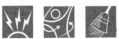

SERVES 6
1½ HOURS

PASTA:

1 box (12 ounces) spaghetti
1 teaspoon salt
1 tablespoon olive oil

1 | Place a 5-quart saucepan filled a little over ⅔ with water over high heat, bring to a boil, and turn down to a low, rolling boil.

2 | Add the 1 teaspoon salt.

3 | Add the spaghetti until it is covered with water.

4 | Cook at a low boil for 8–12 minutes, then, with a pair of tongs, pull one piece of pasta out, let cool, and see if it's still chewy. If it's still a little hard, let cook for 1 more minute and repeat test until it's not fully cooked but no longer hard and chewy.

5 | Remove from the heat, drain, and toss with the olive oil.

SPINACH STUFFING:

2 tablespoons olive oil
1 pound fresh spinach, stemmed
1 small onion coarsely chopped
1 medium leek, thinly sliced
4 garlic cloves, finely chopped
2 teaspoons olive oil (for greasing the bottom
    of the casserole dish)

1 | Place a 5-quart saucepan over medium heat.

2 | Add the 2 tablespoons olive oil, then the remaining ingredients.

3 | Reduce heat to medium-low and cook, stirring, for 10 minutes.

4 | Transfer to a large mixing bowl and set aside.

RICOTTA STUFFING:

1 pound low-fat ricotta cheese

2 whole eggs

1 teaspoon nutmeg

1 tablespoon salt

1 tablespoon ground pepper

1 | Place all the ingredients in a large mixing bowl and mix until well blended.

2 | Add the spinach stuffing and mix with a spoon until combined.

TOPPING:

½ cup grated Parmesan cheese

¼ cup fine bread crumbs

2 tablespoons red chili powder

1 teaspoon salt

1 tablespoon olive oil, drizzled over the top

Blend all the ingredients except the olive oil in a small mixing bowl and set aside.

ASSEMBLY:

1 | Preheat the oven to 350°F.

2 | Grease the bottom of a 9x14-inch casserole dish with the 2 teaspoons of olive oil.

3 | Place the spaghetti and the ricotta mixture in a large mixing bowl and mix until blended.

4 | Fill the prepared casserole dish.

5 | Sprinkle the top evenly with the topping and drizzle with the 1 tablespoon olive oil.

6 | Bake covered for 20 minutes.

7 | Remove the cover and bake an additional 15 minutes.

8 | Remove from the oven and let rest 5 minutes before serving.

Nutrient	Calories (kcal)	Carbohydrates (g)	Protein (g)	Fat (g)
Single Serving	495	55	26	19

Chicken and Legume Stew

   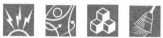

SERVES 4
1½ HOURS

1 pound boneless, skinless chicken breast,
    cut into ½-inch strips
4 cups chicken stock
2 cups cool, clear water
1 can (15 ounces) white beans
½ cup canned chickpeas (garbanzo beans),
    drained
1 onion, chopped into 1-inch pieces
3 garlic cloves, finely chopped

1 | Place all the ingredients in a 4-quart saucepan over high heat until boiling, then lower heat and simmer for 30 minutes.

2 | After simmering, add the following ingredients and simmer for 20 more minutes.

1 pound fresh green beans,
    trimmed and cut into 2-inch pieces
1 cup fresh or frozen and shelled soybeans
½ cup fresh or frozen green peas
1 sprig fresh thyme, or 2 teaspoons dried thyme
1 red bell pepper, cored, seeded,
    and sliced into ½-inch strips
Salt and pepper to taste

JUST BEFORE SERVING:
1 lemon
1 tablespoon olive oil
Pinch salt

1 | With a vegetable peeler, peel the skin off the lemon. Mince finely, then juice half the lemon.

2 | When the stew has finished cooking (50 minutes), add the lemon zest and juice, check the seasonings, and serve hot.

Nutrient	Calories (kcal)	Carbohydrates (g)	Protein (g)	Fat (g)
Single Serving	600	58	56	16

Caramelized Onions

MAKES 4 SERVINGS
15 MINUTES

3 tablespoons olive oil

1 large yellow onion, halved

¼ cup golden raisins

2 tablespoons balsamic vinegar

2 tablespoons brown sugar

1 teaspoon salt

1 | Place a large sauté pan over medium-high heat and add the oil when hot.

2 | Slice each onion half into 5 or 6 lengthwise pieces and add to pan. Reduce the heat to medium or medium-low so the onions cook slowly, not browning or charring.

3 | Stir often until the onions are beginning to turn golden brown.

4 | Add the raisins, balsamic vinegar, brown sugar, and salt.

5 | Stir until all liquid is gone and the onions are deep golden brown, but not charred.

6 | Set aside and keep warm to use in a recipe.

TO SERVE: This is a great flavor add-on for many dishes, including fish, chicken, and steak.

Nutrient	Calories (kcal)	Carbohydrates (g)	Protein (g)	Fat (g)
Single Serving	154	15	1	10

Ancho-Roasted Salmon with Black Beans and Kiwi Sauce

   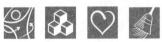

SERVES 4
50 MINUTES

    3 tablespoons olive oil for sauté only

    4 boneless, skinless salmon fillets (6 ounces each)

        (Vegan: Substitute four 4-ounce bricks fresh tofu, patted dry.)

    1 tablespoon freshly squeezed lime juice

    4 tablespoons mesquite honey

    1 tablespoon ancho chili powder or regular red chili powder

    1 teaspoon ground black pepper

    ½ teaspoon salt

1 | Preheat the oven to 400°F.

2 | Warm a large sauté pan over medium-high heat.

3 | Add the oil, wait 1 minute, then add the salmon or tofu.

4 | Sear on one side for 5 minutes, then flip to other side for 1 minute.

5 | Salmon: Roast for 10–20 minutes, or until it begins to flake when tested with a fork. Tofu: Roast for 5–10 minutes, until warmed through.

6 | Place all the remaining ingredients in a small mixing bowl.

7 | Mix together and use to brush onto the salmon (or tofu) when it's finished cooking.

8 | Remove salmon (or tofu) and immediately slather with the ancho-honey mixture.

BLACK BEANS:

    2 15-ounce cans organic black beans, drained

    1 cup vegetable broth or water

    1 garlic clove, minced as finely as possible

    2 tablespoons freshly squeezed orange juice

1 tablespoon unsalted butter

    (Vegan: Substitute olive oil.)

1 teaspoon low-sodium soy sauce

1 tablespoon mesquite honey

Salt and pepper to taste

Place all the ingredients in a 2-quart saucepan over medium heat and simmer uncovered for 30 minutes, until the liquid evaporates.

KIWI SAUCE:

2 kiwifruits, peeled and quartered

3 tablespoons water

1 tablespoon honey

1 teaspoon freshly squeezed lemon juice

Place all the ingredients in a food processor, process until mixture is smooth, and set aside.

TO SERVE: Use the beans as a base and top with salmon or tofu. Spoon kiwi sauce around perimeter of plate.

Nutrient	Calories (kcal)	Carbohydrates (g)	Protein (g)	Fat (g)
Single Serving	449	41	24	21

One-Pot Halibut Stew

SERVES 4
1 HOUR, 25 MINUTES

STEW:

4 cups cool, clear water

1 cup dry white wine

1 head fresh fennel, green tops cut off and set aside and core/root
    removed with a paring knife and thinly sliced

2 medium leeks (white part only), sliced into ¼-inch rings

1 medium onion, thinly sliced

2 garlic cloves, roughly chopped in small pieces

1 sprig fresh thyme

1 pound halibut, skinned and cut into sixteen 1-ounce cubes
    (may also use haddock or whitefish)

8 ounces mussels, rinsed and checked for freshness by pinching the open ones
    (if they don't start closing on their own, toss 'em out)

8 ounces fresh clams, rinsed and checked for freshness

FINISH:

1 medium carrot

2 green onions, cut into ¼-inch rings

1 teaspoon red chili powder

Salt and pepper to taste

GARNISH:

2 tablespoons chopped parsley

1 tablespoon olive oil (for sprinkling on top)

1 tablespoon freshly squeezed lemon juice (for sprinkling on top)

1 Place a 5-quart saucepan over medium-high heat and add all the stew ingredients except for the halibut, mussels, and clams.

2 When the liquid comes to a boil, turn to a low boil and simmer for 10 minutes, add the halibut and cook for 10 minutes, add the clams and cook for 5 minutes, then finally add the mussels and cook for 5 more minutes.

3 With a vegetable peeler, shave ½-inch strips from the carrot.

4 Add the carrot, green onions, chili powder, salt, and pepper, and simmer for 5 additional minutes.

5 Add the garnish ingredients and serve.

Nutrient	Calories (kcal)	Carbohydrates (g)	Protein (g)	Fat (g)
Single Serving	320	22	40	8

Fresh Orange and Coriander Dessert Shake

SERVES 4
10 MINUTES

2 cups plain nonfat yogurt

½ cup nonfat milk

1 pint plain vanilla ice cream

1 orange, peeled and segmented

½ teaspoon vanilla extract

1 teaspoon ground coriander

1 teaspoon ground nutmeg

3 tablespoons honey

1 cup freshly squeezed orange juice

4 mint sprigs, about 4 leaves on each

1 | Place all the ingredients except the orange juice and the mint garnish in a blender and pulse 5 times to begin mixing the ingredients.

2 | Add the orange juice, then purée until smooth.

3 | Pour into tall glasses and garnish with a mint sprig.

Nutrient	Calories (kcal)	Carbohydrates (g)	Protein (g)	Fat (g)
Single Serving	250	40	9	6

Fresh Lime and Mint Dessert Shake

SERVES 4
30 MINUTES

2 cups loosely packed fresh mint leaves

2 cups plain nonfat yogurt

½ cup nonfat milk

1 pint plain vanilla ice cream

1 teaspoon ground coriander

1 tablespoon sugar

4 tablespoons honey

¾ cup freshly squeezed lime juice

¼ cup freshly squeezed orange juice

4 sprigs mint, about 4 leaves on each

1   Place all the ingredients except the lime and orange juices and the mint garnish in a blender and pulse 5 times to begin mixing the ingredients.

2   Add the juices, then purée until smooth.

3   Pour into tall glasses and garnish with a mint sprig.

Nutrient	Calories (kcal)	Carbohydrates (g)	Protein (g)	Fat (g)
Single Serving	258	43	8	6

Frozen Orange Yogurt

SERVES 4
3 HOURS

4 cups plain unsweetened low-fat yogurt

½ cup orange marmalade

2 tablespoons freshly squeezed orange juice

2 tablespoons honey

3 tablespoons cranberry juice

1 Mix all the ingredients except the cranberry juice in a large mixing bowl.

2 Use 4 clean coffee cups.

3 Divide the mixture evenly between the cups.

4 Swirl the cranberry juice on top.

5 Freeze for 3 hours.

Nutrient	Calories (kcal)	Carbohydrates (g)	Protein (g)	Fat (g)
Single Serving	308	55	13	4

Grilled Figs with Lemon Ice Cream and Mint

SERVES 4
40 MINUTES

1 pint vanilla ice cream—if using low-fat,
    add 1 tablespoon honey

2 medium lemons, juiced, seeds discarded

½ medium lemon

2 tablespoons chopped fresh mint

1 tablespoon honey

8 medium figs, ripe and cut in half
    (Can substitute dried figs; soak in warm water
    with 2 tablespoons honey and 1 tablespoon
    brown sugar, drain, and continue recipe.)

4 large mint sprigs, 4 leaves on each

1   Remove pulp from ½ lemon, discard seeds, and set aside.

2   Remove ice cream from freezer to soften for 5–10 minutes.

3   Place the softened ice cream in a large mixing bowl and stir to a creamy consistency.

4   Add the lemon juice, lemon pulp, chopped mint, and honey to the ice cream and stir until mixed in.

5   Place the ice cream back into the freezer for 10 minutes. (This can be done days in advance and served at any time.)

6   Place a medium-size nonstick sauté pan over medium-high heat, or preheat the grill for 10 minutes and clean off with a wire brush.

7 Place the fig halves cut side down on the pan or grill for 2–4 minutes until they are golden in color. Set aside and keep warm. (This can be prepared a day in advance and refrigerated. Rewarm under low broiler for 5 minutes before continuing.)

8 Place a scoop of ice cream and 4 fig halves in each serving bowl and top with a mint sprig.

Nutrient	Calories (kcal)	Carbohydrates (g)	Protein (g)	Fat (g)
Single Serving	188	36	2	4

KEY TO NUTRITION ICONS

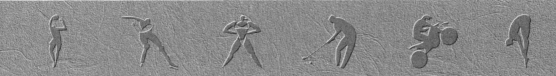

 Firestarter

 Heart-Healthy Fat

 Rapid Replenisher

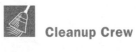 **Cleanup Crew**

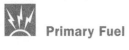 **Primary Fuel**

 Healthy Snack

 Building Block

 Fiber

INDEX

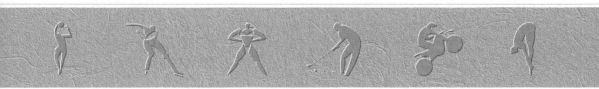

ABOUT THE AUTHORS

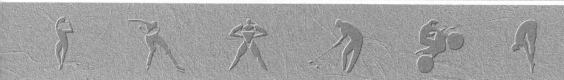

Chris Carmichael is an endurance coach and adviser to Olympic athletes and teams around the world, as well as Lance Armstrong's personal coach. In 1999, Carmichael was named the U.S. Olympic Committee's Coach of the Year. That same year, while guiding Armstrong to his first Tour de France victory, he founded Carmichael Training Systems (CTS) to bring quality coaching to elite athletes and other active people. He is the author of *The Ultimate Ride* and *Food for Fitness*.

Mark Tarbell is the owner of Tarbell's in Phoenix (*Food & Wine* Best Restaurant) and co-owner of The Oven and Home, two restaurants near Denver. He earned his culinary degree at La Varenne and studied wine at the Académie du Vin, both in Paris. Nominated Best Chef—Southwest by the James Beard Foundation, he has cooked at many special events, including one for His Holiness the Dalai Lama. A judge for the L.A. County Fair wine competition and a board member of the International Association of Culinary Professionals'

Culinary Trust, Tarbell is the weekly wine columnist for *The Arizona Republic* and has been published in *Wine & Spirits* and *Food Arts*.

Jim Rutberg has worked with Chris Carmichael and CTS since 1999. He is the coauthor, with Carmichael, of *The Ultimate Ride* and *Food for Fitness*.

Learn more about a limited-time offer of
ONE FREE*MONTH
of CTS Fitness Coaching
by going to

www.foodforfitness.net

Just enter the special promotion code:
foodforfitness
and that's it! It's that easy.
Start your coaching today!

Questions about this offer:
E-mail your questions to: **askcts@trainright.com**

*A one-time registration fee of $4.95 applies to this offer